A Cancer Answer

Holistic BREAST Cancer Management

A Guide to Effective & *Non-Toxic* Treatments

ISBN: 1477490175
ISBN-13: 978-1477490174
Library of Congress Control Number: 2012909105

Cover Art: *Female Silhouette* by Havsekaya / Dreamstime.com

The information in this book is not meant to be diagnostic or
prescriptive. Nor is the information or the book intended to replace
medical advice. The information is offered for information-sharing
purposes and recounts the author's research, personal journey, and
opinions. The contents of this book should not be used as—nor to
give—medical advice, but rather to acquaint readers with what's available
in holistic breast cancer therapies and management, and to share the
author's story of the treatment route she chose for herself, which she
refers to as an "odyssey." If readers choose to consider any information in
this book, the author and publisher assume no responsibilities for readers'
choice(s) or course(s) of action taken, which should be discussed *first with*
readers' physician(s), healthcare practitioner(s), and most definitely *before*
making any decisions regarding any treatment(s) for breast cancer.

Table of Contents

Part I
Understanding Cancer Issues

Part II
Holistic Non-Toxic BREAST Cancer SELF-Management

Following the 'Manufacturer's Manual' That Comes With the Human Body

Part III
Holistic Non-Toxic Healthcare Resources

Acknowledgements

Catherine J Frompovich expressly thanks all whose works have been cited as references, links, and other sources of information, as she respects all authors' works and intellectual property. She hopes to uplift and share intellectual contributions that showcase the fruits of important work by others in the spirit of literary camaraderie, hoping those works may contribute to understanding the issue at hand. It is neither Ms Frompovich's intent nor desire to infringe upon anyone's copyright, as she believes she has used the U.S. Copyright's *Doctrine of Fair Use* equitably and without incurring infringement or plagiarism. All sources are cited in detail and with proper attribution. Thank you to all whose works are cited.

A very special *Thank You* to Dr Buttram, Dr Mejia, Lisa Weir, Dr McCormick, Dr Getson, Liesha Getson, Dr Kracht, Dr Laibow, and Dr Jordan for your extra-special contributions. Without a doubt, readers certainly will appreciate your input. Thanks again.

Lastly, I cannot forget the Design Team at CreateSpace. You took all my ideas that I envisioned for the book and made them into the reality it is. I appreciate you.

Dedication

To females everywhere

May you never experience the mental, emotional, and physical torments that accompany a breast cancer diagnosis.

But, if you should, I hope this book can help you sort out what's possible.

As the Reverend Martin Luther King once said, ***"To solve a problem, you got to get your mind right."***

Inspiration From the Ages & the Sages

A wise man should consider that health is the greatest of human blessings, and learn how by his own thought to derive benefit from his illnesses.

... Hippocrates (c.460 BCE-370BCE)
Regimen in Health

Follow nature, and she will be your instructor. The ways of nature are simple, and she does not require any complicated prescriptions. The invisible forces in the body are powerful and may be guided by the imagination and propelled by the will.

... Paracelsus (1493-1541)
One of the greatest physicians of all time

Most men die of their remedies, not of their illnesses.

... Moliere (1622-1673)
French playwright

Doctors give drugs of which they know little, into bodies, of which they know less, for diseases of which they know nothing at all.

... Voltaire (1694-1778)
French philosopher/Historian

The doctor of the future will give no medication, but will interest his patients in the care of the human frame, diet and in the cause and prevention of disease.

... Thomas A Edison (1847-1931)
American scientist/Inventor

Since the human body tends to move in the direction of its expectations—plus or minus—it is important to know that attitudes of confidence and determination are no less a part of the treatment program than medical and science technology.

... Norman Cousins (1915-1990)
American journalist/Professor

The estimated total number of iatrogenic deaths—that is, deaths induced inadvertently by a physician or surgeon or by medical treatment or diagnostic procedures— in the US annually is 783,936.......while 553,251 died of cancer.

... Gary Null, PhD, et al. "Death By Medicine" (1945—)
Complementary/Alternative Medicine advocate/Author

Foreword

Harold E Buttram, MD
Board Certified, Environmental Medicine

Having written several papers with Catherine Frompovich, I've come to know and respect her knowledge about the human body and its interaction with the environment and, more precisely, how Catherine respects the role of food and nutrition in health and wellness.

Since Catherine matriculated in holistic modalities and natural nutrition she has great reverence for the body's inborn ability regarding life processes, particularly its ability to heal disease when given proper guidance and modalities. Nothing exemplifies that principle more, in her opinion, than the body's ability to heal itself of breast cancer without toxic modalities.

During Catherine's studies that led to advanced degrees in Nutrition and Holistic Health Sciences and a Certification in Orthomolecular Theory and Practice, she realized and has valued how important it is to follow the "owner's manual" that comes with the human body—Nature's intended way of life, living, and healthcare.

Catherine spent numerous years in practice as a consulting *natural* nutritionist. She had an enviable reputation that even medical doctors recognized when, in fact, they would send their patients to her with the endorsement, "I can't help you, but Catherine will be able to."

Catherine made recommendations that changed lifestyle and diets, something way ahead of its time—that was all she did—and the rest is history, as they say. Now that she's retired, she still has former clients sending her thank you notes. Catherine takes no credit. She contends they got well because of what a person does to work within the framework that God and Nature provide, not what toxic chemicals in air, food, and water destroy. Catherine displays a similar "ahead of the curve thinking" as others have in medical history.

Ignaz Semmelweis was an Austrian obstetrician who practiced his profession at a birthing center in Vienna in the mid-nineteenth century, a time and place where maternity death rates were an appalling 30 percent from "childbed fever," due to poor sanitary conditions and practices of the times. Semmelweis observed that medical students would perform autopsies on the victims of childbed fever and then often go to maternity wings and deliver babies without washing their hands. Deeply troubled about the losses at the birthing center, it occurred to him that the students could be carrying some noxious substance on their hands to the mothers in the delivery wards. Acting upon this intuitive impression, he mandated that no doctor should touch a woman in labor without first washing his hands in the rather harsh soap of the times. As a result the mortality rate in his wing soon dropped from 30 to 3 percent, while other wings continued with their usual 30 percent mortalities. In spite of this epoch-making contribution, his work was ignored, and he became ostracized by his colleagues and remained so until his death.

In the field of nutrition, the story of Archie Kalokerinos, an Australian health officer who worked among the Australian aborigines in the 1960s and 1970s, is quite similar. When he first began his work, Kalokerinos similarly became appalled by a 50 percent infant mortality that was taking place. Noting signs of scurvy among some of the infants and observing that many deaths took place following immunizations, especially if ill with a viral-type illness, Kalokerinos began administering vitamin C supplements, improving their diets, and avoiding vaccines during viral-type illnesses (even if just a runny nose). Subsequently the infant death rate dropped from 50 percent to 3 percent in his district.

It is entirely possible that Kalokerinos himself did not recognize the full scope of his findings as concerns body inflammation, now known to be associated with Alzheimer's disease, coronary heart disease, and cancer. It should be stressed that inflammation, in and of itself, is a healing process that always follows tissue injury whether from physical trauma, pathogenic microbes, or toxic chemicals, the latter now almost certainly becoming predominant due to the prevalence of toxic environmental chemicals in air, food, and water. It is quite likely that, with the passage of time, the pioneer work of Kalokerinos will come to be recognized with the same honor and stature as that now held for Semmelweis, because antioxidants provide comparable protection from harmful chemicals as soap and boiling water do for dangerous microbes.

Antioxidants play a more important role in health and well being, but apparently are treated as 'stepchildren' by the medical profession. In *Exodus* of the Old Testament, we are told how God provided "manna" as food for the Israelites, on which they thrived as long as they followed what had been provided for them. Based on what is now known, it is a virtual certainty that manna was abundantly supplied with antioxidants as a universal protection against disease-causing toxins. Most people today are familiar with the antioxidant vitamins A, C, and E, but there are also many other antioxidants.

For many years the C-reactive protein blood test, a nonspecific test for body inflammation, has been used as a risk factor for coronary heart disease. Of special interest in this area is a report in *Townsend Letter* on "Arterial Scurvy" by Thomas E Levy in which the author maintains that the coronary arteries remain resistant to deposits of calcium, cholesterol, and other lipids until the connective tissue of the arteries begins crumbling from vitamin C deficiency (scurvy), since the formation of connective tissue is dependent on vitamin C. Levy also wrote:

> *"Arguably the most intriguing and fascinating aspect of vitamin C is that it serves as the ultimate antidote. Depending on the nature of the toxin and the timing of vitamin C administration, vitamin C can serve as a chemical, mechanical, and/or physiologic antidote.... The literature clearly establishes this ability of vitamin C to clinically resolve the*

syndrome of poisoning associated with a large and diverse array of toxins."

Recently the C-reactive protein blood test was found to have a new application in the *Pourcyrous study* in which 239 preterm infants were subjected to single and multiple vaccines at < two months age in a hospital intensive care unit followed by C-reactive blood tests which reported abnormal elevations in 85 percent administered multiple vaccines and 70 percent of those administered a single vaccine. Although the Pourcyrous study does not tell us the source of the inflammation, the facts that 17 percent of those receiving single vaccines experienced intraventricular brain hemorrhages, and those receiving mixed vaccines had 24 percent intraventricular brain hemorrhages, and that, overall, 16 percent had potentially lethal cardiorespiratory events (the cardiorespiratory control center is located in a lower area of the brain), it is a near certainty that the elevations in C-reactive blood tests represented brain inflammation.

In a fascinating study entitled, "C-reactive protein concentration and concentrations of blood vitamins, carotenoids, and selenium among United States adults," it was found that C-reactive protein levels varied inversely and significantly associated with concentrations of (antioxidants including) retinol, retinyl esters, vitamin C, *alpha* carotene, *beta* carotene, cryptoxanthine, lutein/zeaxanthin, lycopene, and selenium. **These findings suggest that the inflammatory process, through the production of reactive oxygen species, may deplete stores of antioxidants.** In other words, the implications are that antioxidants, as a single variant—whether by diet and/

or supplementation—are significantly protective against cancer, heart disease, the leading killers of our times, as well as Alzheimer's disease.

In spite of the historic and scientific evidence outlined above, mainstream medicine has not shown any *serious* interest in more than cursory or token use of antioxidants.

In closing, the subject of antioxidants has been chosen for the *Foreword* as representative for each of the chapters in this remarkable book, which provides guidelines for those seeking "*natural*" approaches for treatment of breast cancer, which undoubtedly will stand the tests of time and must be considered seriously if the war on cancer is to be won.

Harold E Buttram, MD

Introduction

Catherine's Story

OMG! It hit my psyche like a nine-point-zero earthquake, tsunami, and tornado *combined.* OMG, what do I do now? That was my honest reaction to a physician confirming that there was a mass in my right breast, and I was being steered into quick action to deal with it. All of a sudden, it seemed life had dumped a ton-and-a-half of lemons on me and I was seeking some way to crawl out from under to make lemonade.

Being inclined toward a holistic lifestyle most of my life and having earned degrees in Nutrition and Holistic Health Sciences, I had to evaluate—and re-evaluate—what was being suggested: mammograms, biopsy, surgery, radiation, chemo-therapy, *tamoxifen*—the whole nine yard standard allopathic treatment for breast cancer. So what did I do? I went within and prayed. I'm not ashamed to admit that I asked Creator God and His ever-helpful Angels for guidance to know what to do and have the courage and commitment to follow through.

What I was not told in the rather *must do* allopathic regi-men, were the damaging side effects of *tamoxifen* [1], which I knew. Furthermore, a Swedish study linked *tamoxifen* to other cancers. Dr Janette D Sherman, MD, has this to say in Chapter 9 of her book, *Life's Delicate Balance,* about the standard breast cancer drug:

Between 1970 and 1987, more than 3 million women were administered tamoxifen for a cumulative time of more than 5.8 million patient years! Unfortunately, except for specific clinical trials, few records have been kept on women given the drug.[2] To which I say, "Why, and what does that mean?"

Every allopathic standard modality offered as cancer treatment was anathema to my very belief, lifestyle, and former resolve that if I ever were confronted with a cancer scare, I'd go the holistic route. Now was the "rubber hitting the road" time and I could not tarry nor make a mistake in my choice of treatment.

Since I'm a consumer healthcare researcher and a retired healthcare professional who networks with medical doctors, researchers, and PhDs around the globe, I confided in some and received such feedback that I was overwhelmed by the responses insofar as my wanting to go the holistic treatment route. I cannot tell you how much research data was offered— a lot of which I was aware—and how affirming it was for me to hear that my choice was the one that would get me well and not compromise my immune system further or contribute to secondary cancers.

Both my parents died of cancer: Mom, breast; Dad, stomach. Were heredity and genes playing a role in what was going on in my right breast? Personally, "I did not want to go there," as I thought it was not necessary and I wasn't playing the blame game. However, I did acknowledge that in my past I had been poisoned, perhaps, on two separate occasions—years apart—by unscrupulous individuals making illegal substances, possibly methamphetamines, and venting or flushing them, which created toxic fumes coming into our house. The second time airborne fumes almost killed me, and I believe they did kill my late husband, who was twenty-four years older than I. He had contracted emphysema from the first bout of being exposed to whatever those toxic fumes were.

Years before those exposures I also had been exposed to formaldehyde in carpeting we had installed in the first house we purchased. Unbeknown to us—as to most people in the early 1970s—wall-to-wall carpeting was full of formaldehyde that did a number on my immune system and led to my earning degrees in holistic health sciences. So, having had my turn in the barrel at least three times, I began to realize that the true culprit was man-made-chemicals exacting their latent tolls, so why should I add more chemicals to my body through conventional allopathic breast cancer treatment, e.g., chemotherapy and ionizing radiation. My decision was I'm going holistic, and so I did.

That's when a true odyssey began and one that I must say, I'm enjoying. It's taken me down pathways and into so much knowledge that I cannot express how thankful I am to those who have been there and documented what worked for them. However, that information is not readily available and is scorned with inquisition-like zeal by the medical and pharmaceutical establishments that control the politics of healthcare—and cancer treatment, in particular—in the United States.

I must confess that, upon the insistence of the holistic physician I chose to work with, I went for evaluation to a breast surgeon the doctor recommended, which turned out to be a turn-off event for me. Ironically, I was there on my 73rd birthday. The staff sang happy birthday to me as I walked from the waiting room into the private consultation room. Although the breast surgeon was professional in every way, I was not impressed by what I perceived as 'fear tactics' to get going immediately, if not sooner, with allopathic treatment. All I could do was hold my tongue, secretly pray for getting out of there without making a commitment, and getting on with what I wanted for *MY* right breast and body.

Admittedly, I felt totally relieved after the surgeon's consultation that I had made the correct decision for me. It was like ten tons of fear were lifted off my mind, heart, and soul. I was free to be me and get the best care that I knew would not be toxic and heal my body rather than tear it down from all the chemical intervention they had to offer. I happen to be a person who cannot handle pharmaceutical medicines from childhood—a flu vaccine in 1957 almost killed me—so I've learned how to take care of my body without chemical intervention, going the natural route. Even when my late husband and I were poisoned by toxins, I/we went the homeopathic, natural route and got well. Now this. Why?

Being one who needs to understand the whys in life, I prayed for an answer to that annoying question. When I get hold of an issue, I don't let go until I'm satisfied that I have the correct answer. I got my answer in the form of a dream wherein I was writing a book about my treatment, which I'm doing right here. The other was what I'd call paranormal experiences while undergoing acupuncture.

Before I tell you about that, let me share that within two days of seeing the surgeon, I had five days of acupuncture at the capable hands of a gifted Chinese acupuncturist who, I believe, really jump-started my immune system into high-gear response.

During the third treatment, I was laying face down with needles stuck all over the backside of my entire body—head to toe. I now know what it feels like to be a pincushion. Shortly before the session ended, I recall that I was interacting with someone/thing/entity in the room and I can remember vividly saying, "Please don't go; don't leave me alone. I want to go with you." To which I heard the distinct reply as clearly as anything, "No, you have to stay." I was in total shock or disbelief, to say the least. Where did that voice come from; who was it; was it real? It took me almost an hour to calm down after that experience. I felt like I had been zapped with a stun gun. My body tingled; my brain froze; I functioned like an android. Driving home I began to realize that there was another dimension to what I was going through and that I was being directed in a way that would be most helpful, as I truly believe in, "Ask and you shall receive; seek and you shall find; knock and it shall be opened to you." I was doing all those things and answers were starting to come to me.

Since acupuncture was the very first holistic regimen I embarked on, I think you ought to know that I experienced two other affirmations—at least to the way I think—that I had chosen the correct treatment regimen for me. One was the second treatment at the acupuncturist when I went to the restroom, it was occupied, so I had to wait. The person coming out the door amazed me. A Buddhist monk in saffron robes, sandals, and wooden beads around his neck and wrist, started to walk past me, then backed up and bowed deeply to me. I acknowledged his bow with a bow of my head. When I got inside the restroom I blurted, *"Yes! I hear you talkin' to me."*

The third paranormal encounter I had was while I was reclining on my back with needles in the front side of my body preparing to relax after having said prayers for healing to be activated in my body's meridians through the needles, I closed my eyes to rest and there before me was the face of the Master and Lord Jesus Christ. Wow! What an affirmation, I thought. Can it get any better than that? Here I was on the very first leg of my holistic cancer treatment odyssey and I'm getting what I can only feel are positive affirmations that I'm on the right track. And so, I didn't look back and proceeded full throttle ahead into further researching and taking holistic treatments. As I write this, the tumor is breaking up, and I pray it will be gone in no time. *Belief is a most important aspect to healing.*

This book may not be for every female who is searching for the correct modality to treat her breast cancer problem, and I respect that. However, for me, all that I've researched over the years—and particularly now at this critical time in my life— has led to and confirmed my resolve that I was doing the most natural thing I could possibly do to heal not only my breast, but my entire body, since cancer really is systemic. After all, healing is a Creator-given, built-in process within our body's physiological makeup. If you cut your finger, doesn't it heal?

After much soul-searching, prayer, and interaction with many medical doctors, nurses, and others whose expertise I highly respect, I came to the realization that what I had to do was to make certain that in my mind I was positive I could live with the decision. One cannot play hopscotch-therapy protocol with such a diagnosis.

One of the most influential aspects in my decision making processes revolved around just how sick I wanted to become, since I know the ramifications of radiation and chemotherapy—they are immediate and long range. Here I was functioning on all cylinders, working to midnight most nights, feeling no pain nor discomfort, so I rationalized that if I were to be sick, I'd rather be sick at the very end and not suffer the ravages of hell for numerous years, no matter how short or long they would be from radiation and/or chemotherapy. I know of numerous persons who have gone the conventional 'cut-burn-poison' route, as many call it, and after several years into their protocol having gone through numerous rounds of agonizing treatments with radiation, chemotherapy, losing their hair, extreme edema and nausea, they then learn that they have secondary cancers or there are metastases. So how is that a cure?

For me that was not an option, since I don't regard a 'supposed cure' that is worse than the original disease—or a protocol that gives you secondary health problems, e.g., secondary cancers sooner or later—the correct approach to healthcare *for me.* I cannot understand or process within my intelligence how subjecting body tissues to ionizing nuclear radiation doesn't cause added harm, either short or long term. Many folks suffer from radiation sickness and burns, something many patients experience but are not told about upfront. That was not an option for me. [3]

Personally, I question the efficacy of horrendously poisonous chemotherapy drugs—many fluoride-based—and their catastrophic tolls on vital organs such as liver, lungs, heart, and most of all, the brain, since many chemo drugs inadvertently do cross the blood brain barrier. A good number of folks who take chemotherapy suffer with depression, something I didn't want to deal with because depression then would be induced in me by pharmacology—an iatrogenic [doctor caused] illness, since I'm not a person who gets depressed. Who needs depression in addition to all the other side effects of chemo, I rationalized.

The downside of conventional breast cancer treatments left very little in the way of hope *for me,* since my own mother died of it while under conventional cancer treatment. To my way of thinking, there is so much that needs revamping in conventional breast cancer treatment, specifically fortifying the immune system and nutritionally revitalizing the entire body. Allopathic medicine just "doesn't go there" adequately, in my opinion as a retired *natural* nutritionist. The proof for my making that statement can be found in hospitals after breast—or any surgery—check out the meals hospitals provide cancer patients. That to me is a total health putdown, a disregard, and an insult to the intelligence of the human body's ability to recover when given proper nutritional support and non-toxic therapies. The human body has been functioning for thousands of years on its own, as we who are alive today are testimonials to its capability to live, thrive, reproduce, and survive. But we must remember—no one gets off the planet alive.

As a consumer healthcare researcher for thirty-five years and counting, and a retired *natural* nutritionist who matriculated in *natural* nutrition—how food is handled in the body and its interactions for health and well being—I keep thinking about the philosophical differences between allopathic medicine and holistic healthcare and how each regards the cause of disease, which probably is the genuine driving force in my thinking.

Allopathic conventional medicine, based in pharmacology and vaccinology, i.e., prescription drugs and vaccines, believes in and practices the *germ theory* of illness, whereas holistic healthcare believes in and practices the *terrain theory*, or *biological terrain* theory, espoused by Antoine Beauchamp (1816-1908), which corrects body biochemistry by fortifying it with nutrients, not horrendous—often toxic—chemicals.

Louis Pasteur (1822-1895) fashioned the germ theory, i.e., dangerous germs attacking us and causing disease. Beauchamp, his contemporary, claimed that germs could not do anything to cause disease unless the *body's internal environment* [biological terrain] was unhealthy, biochemically out of balance and thus a suitable environment for disease to establish itself. To understand that concept, please consider a petri cell culture dish. For a culture to grow, everything—growth medium, temperature, spore or specimen—has to be favorable or you won't get results.

According to a deathbed confession of sorts, Pasteur was said to have agreed that Beauchamp's theory of disease was correct.

"Bernard was right; the pathogen is nothing; the terrain is everything."

… Louis Pasteur's deathbed words (September 28, 1895)

There's an entertaining analogy about the two theories of disease as portrayed via a cartoon spoof "The Town of Allopath," created by Mercola.com and available online at <mercola.com/townofallopath/index.htm>.[4]

Needless to say, we have to ask ourselves what role does our toxic lifestyle today play in the inordinate occurrences of cancers, and breast cancer in particular. Our grandmothers and great grandmothers weren't plagued with it. To my way of thinking, Beauchamp was correct and so was Pasteur, to a point. Why do I say that?

My opinion on that is there's a middle ground factor almost comparable to the pH bar of acid/alkaline balance. My reasoning is: There truly are germs and microorganisms; the microscope proved that. If you really want to see what's rattling around in your blood, examine it using a dark field microscope.

Human biochemistry and our immune system are our inner environment—*terrain*—and just like every vibratory entity, it and we must live within specialized environments whether it is personal, local, community, national, global, or even cosmic.

To support that statement consider that astronauts must use specialized spacesuits to travel out of our usual gravity field, oxygen-rich, and gamma-radiation-free environment. If they didn't have an artificially created environment in which to breathe and function, they'd get sick, be non-functional, and/or die. So one's environment—terrain as Beauchamp claimed—*is* key to health, maintaining it, and functioning optimally.

The problem as I assess it is that one philosophical approach—allopathy's germ theory—wants to dominate and control healthcare treatments to the exclusion of the equally valid holistic—biological terrain. That's why healthcare costs are skyrocketing while humans are getting sicker, especially with cancer and other chronic diseases. There needs to be more integration and implementation of biochemistry regarding our inner terrain rather than toxic pharmacology in medicine for more effective results, I think.

Those who know me—friends and colleagues—feel that my writing a book about *holistic breast cancer treatment* is the best thing I can do to help others understand options and their ability to regain health, plus informing others that there just may be "better mousetraps" out there to deal with it. As they say, "Been there, done that" and "Walk the talk" establishes a credibility factor. Didn't the Greek philosopher Plato state that the reality of our world could only be known through our experiences? So that's why I'm sharing with you what I've learned—nothing like experience, something few medical doctors actually know about; they just go with the toxic chemical protocols they were taught about by pharmaceutical company sales representatives.

Holistic breast cancer treatment(s) may not be for you, but if you want to know what it's about, how it works or is worked, and uncover resources, I hope this book will help you find the strength and peace in coming to a decision—which ever it may be—plus a cure in the treatment and management of breast cancer.

Perhaps you would like to know that after seven weeks using holistic breast cancer management/treatment, my haircutter said to me during my monthly haircut, "Catherine, what's going on with you? Your hair is getting darker in the back and the gray you had at your temples is almost gone! I've never seen anyone grow dark hair back from gray. What's going on?"

My answer to Angela was, "I guess my holistic breast cancer treatment and nutritional program have revved up my body chemistry to grow new and healthy cells." Angela's reply was, "Unbelievable—who would have thought?" Personally, I've known it all along and so do many others going back to Beauchamp. However, that information is deliberately embargoed from the public by vested interests, I truly believe, and that's why I want to share such a personal story.

For my part, I think the war on cancer has been fought far too long and needs to be won. Cancer in some form affects one in every two men and one in every three women in the United States. According to *BreastCancer.org* statistics, besides skin cancer, breast cancer is the most commonly diagnosed cancer among U.S. women. More than 1 in 4 cancers in women (about 28%) are breast cancer. [5]

Cancer battlegrounds seem to be expanding beyond our ability to contain the disease. Can that be from treatment toxicity, secondary cancers, or plain ineffectiveness, despite hyped survival statistics? It seems that after all these years of the "same old, same old" surgery-radiation-chemotherapy modalities, standard cancer battle plans need to be changed to more humane—*holistic*—treatment with certainly more effective modalities other than the average-costing $111,000 *a year* chemotherapy protocol. With that kind of money involved, chemotherapy is very cost effective for the pharmaceutical industry and, in my opinion, is a probable and valid reason there just may be no incentive to win the war on cancer.

Many health insurers are deciding NOT to cover *new Avastin®* prescriptions—a drug that blocks angiogenesis [the growth of new blood vessels] for conventional treatment of breast cancer patients. Effective October 17, 2011, breast cancer patients insured by Blue Shield of California will be searching for ways and means to deal with managing and curing the disease. This book ought to help women separate the *"wheat from the chaff"* when it comes to dealing with breast cancer modalities that will block angiogenesis through diet and other holistic means.

This paragraph you are reading now is being written on a most auspicious day, October 12, 2011. I had my second six-week checkup with the holistic physician managing my case and received exceptionally good and exciting news. The two tumors in my right breast have decreased in size between 25 and 30 percent in the twelfth week of being on my holistic breast cancer treatment protocol. I will continue documenting the progress in the *Introduction* until the book is finished.

However, I feel that cancer may be compared to the dreaded disease of biblical times—leprosy or Hansen's disease—that apparently struck folks so often, even to the point of being cited in gospel stories about Jesus curing ten lepers. Back then poor personal sanitation and nutrition, along with human waste pollution apparently were rampant, which compromised the immune system of genetically prone individuals.

Today a comparable analogy, I think, is cancer in all its forms, as cancer results from the *ultimate biological insult* to body chemistry from chemical pollution in food, water, and air, plus radioactive fission particle vapors from the nuclear power industry venting daily into the atmosphere. Chemtrails— those crisscross patterns in the skies sprayed from planes—rain down upon us horrendous chemicals and fine particles of neurotoxic aerosolized aluminum [6], plus other toxins that need to be added to the cancer equation, I have come to believe.

Before I end my *Introduction*, I'd like to share with you that I have tried to document as much information as possible with *Endnotes* that you will find at the back of the book. The book contains numerous references to online Internet websites, which I thought could help you understand what I was discussing. However, I'd like to caution you that some Internet search engines are not recognizing some URL addresses and may say "Error Page" or something similar. Often I experienced that only to find that when I placed the URL into the Google search engine, lo and behold, Google found it. Just like anything else in life, and also with cancer treatments, there are alternative ways to doing things.

There's one central and essential message I'd like to leave you with and it is: This book is not an indictment of allopathic medicine; it's a critique documenting one individual's experiences over decades of having "fallen through the cracks" of the allopathic health paradigm, not finding help, and too many times having suffered with serious adverse reactions to its 'muse', pharmacology, which mandated that I find another way to health and wellness. Gratefully, I found it in holistic healthcare and have thrived.

Let me leave this with you to consider, which I hope will encourage you, too, to stretch your mind. What I cite next I wrote in the 1980s: *During the course of time and with the advancement of various sciences, several different means of measurement and standards have evolved—all accurate and acceptable within today's system of socio-economics and every day living practices. So, too, can there be different approaches to health and wellness.*

There's the metric system. Once we used to say freezing was 32ºF (Fahrenheit). Now we can say freezing is 0ºC (Celsius) and still be correct.

USA travels on the mileage system whereas most of the world goes by kilometers.

Who is to deny music its system of graphs, symbols and special language? Only those who have studied music can read, write or play music. Those who don't understand it are confused by its strange looking hieroglyphics.

There's a long ton and a short ton. There's standard time and daylight saving time.

There are several weight standards: avoirdupois, troy, apoth-ecaries, U.S. liquid measures, and U.S. dry measure, British im-perial liquid and dry measures.

There should be more than allopathic medicine to legally use as a healthcare system in the USA.

I hope and trust by writing this book and sharing what I've done during my breast treatment odyssey, I can help women realize that there *are* effective, non-toxic treatments and man-agement for breast cancer, and that life can become cancer-free without horrendous chemicals and ionizing radiation. I know—because I've taken that route.

May the Light of Creator God be your Guide. I wish you abounding wellness and joy.

Catherine J Frompovich
May 2012

Part I
Understanding Cancer Issues

"Unless we put medical freedom into the Constitution, the time will come when medicine will organize into an undercover dictatorship to restrict the art of healing to one class of men and deny equal privileges to others."

Benjamin Rush, MD
Signer, the U.S. Declaration of Independence 1776

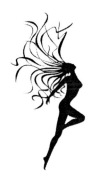

Chapter One
Why Do Humans Get Sick?

Every individual organism that has a distinctive genetic background has distinctive nutritional needs, which must be met for optimal well being.

… Roger J Williams (1893—1988)
American biochemist/Pioneer nutrition researcher

*B*efore we talk about breast cancer—or any type of cancer—maybe we ought to look into why we get sick in the first place, and cancer in particular.

As far as I can ascertain, humans have been on Planet Earth for thousands of years, possibly closer to one hundred thousand years, maybe more, during which time they—and we their progeny—have evolved into sentient beings with specific life-sustaining needs of air, water, food, shelter, and companionship.

After decades of debate, paleoanthropologists now agree the genetic and fossil evidence suggests that the modern human species – Homo sapiens – evolved in Africa between 100,000 and 200,000 years ago.[7]

There's scientific and archeological evidence that humans lived and thrived on the North American continent about 50,000 years ago. Fossils and other ancient artifacts confirm *Homo erectus/sapiens* presence and lifestyles in China and other landmasses on Earth's ever-active tectonic plates, including dramatic weather patterns and climate changes ranging from ice ages to the great Noah flood to desertification of previously viable lands. Despite such conditions, humans still thrived, survived, and multiplied.

There is an amazing video documenting a 12,000-year-old civilization that apparently thrived at Göbekli Tepe, Turkey.[8] Please visit this website <forbiddenknowledgetv.com/videos/ancient-civilizations/12000-year-old-stone-structures.html>.

During that extensive timeline lifestyles progressed from rudimentary gatherer/hunters to a self-sufficient agrarian standard of living that lasted, for the most part, until the beginning of the 20th century, and progressed into what now we consider sophisticated and high tech living. Humans went from building a fire at the cave entrance to keep out wild and ferocious animals to building communal ramparts and moats to today's electronic surveillance mechanisms that notify someone else—usually a monitoring system or police—that intruders are breaking into homes, offices, and public buildings.

Some would say, we've come a long way, let's keep on going.

That encapsulated version of human existence omits one apparently important aspect of human evolution: health, especially since there were no medical doctors, pharmaceutical companies, or medical interventions that we have today. So how did they make it? Luck? Chance? Or is it something else? That something else very well could have been their ability to live close to the land from which they gathered their sustenance.

Today, according to U.S. EPA demographics, less than 1 percent of the U.S. population claims farming as an occupation, while less than 2 percent actually live on farms. That means humans have lost the ability to grow and produce their food—the key to health—consequently depending upon Big Agra and industrial farmers for food and nutritional sustenance, the food processing industry, which further negates nutrient content with chemically-synthesized edibles, plus the ever-present fast food industry.

Getting back to our genetic ancestors, one has to wonder and also question how their health fared despite all the medical spin we hear today about modern medicine keeping us alive and well. So how did they really make it? For starters, they evolved with Nature and natural elements that did not impede nor hinder DNA nor damage its telomeres, thereby allowing humans to pass on genetic information that apparently was robust and healthy, especially during the earliest times when humans ate what is theorized as the "caveman diet." [9]

As farfetched as such a dietary scheme may seem, it is the most viable food paradigm since the art of *haute cuisine*, which apparently had its genesis when Catherine de' Medici married King Henry II of France in the mid 1500s and brought her Italian chefs with her to France, thereby instituting a stylized cuisine later known as French cooking that to this day is prized as the epitome of the culinary arts.

The caveman diet logically consisted of edibles the gatherer-hunter lifestyle generated as dietary food staples, most of which were eaten raw, e.g., fruits, nuts, seeds, root and green vegetables, and later in time, cooked pulses [lentils and beans that the Bible talks about in Genesis 25]. Manioc, or cassava root, to this day is a dietary staple in many parts of the globe.

The caveman diet's apparent dietary mainstay—raw foods—provided optimum nutritional value from enzymes, those powerful biochemical catalysts that energize life sustaining forces and systems in the human body. Since raw food enzymes are inactivated and/or destroyed at 118 degrees Fahrenheit, cooking—unless using quick blanching—provides very little raw food enzymes. They are the powerhouses that kept our ancient ancestors well and thriving, apparently without the professionals most folks today cannot seem to live—or so they think—medical doctors.

Another most important nutritional aspect of the caveman diet was the inordinate amount of minerals that it supplied and, in particular, potassium, which is to soft body tissue what calcium is to bone. Furthermore, that caveman diet most likely provided a critical and balanced ratio of sodium to potassium for maximum cellular viscosity and tension. Today's modern diet is overwhelmed with sodium molecules used in additives, preservatives, and other food preparation and enhancing chemicals in addition to sodium chloride, table salt.

If ancient humans ate meat, that practice may not have been very often because they first had to hunt, catch, kill, and prepare it for consumption, i.e., remove fur and skin—laborious tasks. Chickens and eggs in the human diet in China can be traced back as far as 6,000 BCE. One nutritional aspect about animal protein, though, is certain: Animals consumed back then as food were *grass-fed* animals browsing on grasses, thereby providing optimum nutrient payloads in their milks and meats, not like today's cattle fed soy and corn, most of which is genetically modified that includes toxins from inordinate amounts of pesticide sprays used in growing GMO crops used as cattle feed and silage—and humans, too, in cereals, breads, and most processed foods.

That switch from *grass-fed to grain-fed* animals most likely precipitated problems within the gut and intestinal tracts of cattle, who by Nature were designed to be grazers, not force-fed grain guzzlers. It is highly probable that, that switch has reprogrammed the intestinal flora in cattle that today, along with high rations of prophylactic antibiotics, may be causing many issues with e-coli in meat products. Science even came up with *cannulated* cows—cows with windows in their stomachs—to figure out what's going on with cows' nutritional status. The answer is very simple: Industrial dairy farming changed how the cow eats from its natural ages-old diet of grass to one of grains that apparently is giving cows allergic reactions that, in turn, create intestinal flora problems in tandem with adverse effects from the genetically-modified bovine growth hormone [bST] injected daily to produce more milk, which basically causes mastitis in cow udders along with pus in their milk.

In 1991 Otzi the Iceman's preserved body was found protruding from an Italian Alpine glacier where he had perished at least 5,000 years ago, according to radiocarbon testing. Scientists performed all types of tests on his remains and found

The Iceman's stomach held cultivated wheat, possibly consumed as bread; game meat, and dried sloe plums. [10]

The sloe plum is similar to today's Damson plum, but very bitter in taste.

However, an extremely late autopsy found that Otzi had a disease condition, arthritis. He apparently had been murdered, as there were trauma marks on his body and what appeared to be an arrow in his shoulder. That unfortunate finding sadly indicates violence also has been a lifestyle trait for millennia.

As humans progressed along the timeline of life and living, food played an integral part in their development. In the Old Testament of the Bible, we find this pointed directive:

God said, "I have given you every plant with seeds on the face of the earth and every tree that has fruit with seeds. This will be your food." Genesis 1:29

In the *Book of Psalms,*

He causes the grass to grow for the cattle, and herb for the service of man: that he may bring forth food out of the earth. Psalm 104:14

Note that it says *grass*, not soy or corn.

Regarding the consumption of meat,

You are therefore to make a distinction between the clean animal and the unclean, and between the unclean bird and the clean; and you shall not make yourselves detestable by animal or by bird or by anything that creeps on the ground, which I have separated for you as unclean. Leviticus 20:25

The Mosaic Law diet goes back four thousand years and is set forth in the Old Testament books *Leviticus, Numbers,* and *Deuteronomy.* It's said that during the Israelites bondage in Egypt they gained a taste for the produce there, namely onions and some herbs. During their years in the desert, they rebelled against Moses at times because they did not have those delicious foods they had been accustomed to eating.

It seems the *Mosaic Law* dietary became a way of life that expanded upon the caveman diet insofar as progressing with humans to include other foods plus culinary regimes that were required for health and food safety since there was no refrigeration, plus the lack of proper sanitation. Those dietary requirements must have been successful, since nowhere in the Bible do we find that the ancient Hebrews suffered mass food poisonings or food-induced illnesses. We read about famines, leprosy, and other issues but don't seem to find food sicknesses *per se* that should have been reported if such things either were commonplace or disastrous—many people dying from food issues. Nonetheless, I was able to find an interesting article online titled *"Bible ills and remedies"* by JR Gwilt, PhD, published in the *Journal of the Royal Society of Medicine*, December 1986, that you just may want to read, as I found it rather informative. [11]

One food and dietary anomaly the Bible apparently does not address is the present day industrial farming practices that impact and dramatically alter chemical and nutritional compositions of foods derived from animals, particularly dairy cows. Consider this: prophylactic antibiotics in cattle feed along with other drugs to treat udder mastitis in cows that occurs with more frequency because of daily injections of bST or *Bovine Somatotropin*.

Now, the new science of biotechnology makes it possible to work with DNA, the part of a cell that contains the genetic information for an animal or a plant. Scientists have determined which gene in cattle controls or codes for the production of bST. They have removed this gene from cattle and inserted it into a bacterium called Escherichia coli. *This bacterium, which is found in the intestinal tract of humans and animals, acts like a tiny factory and produces large amounts of bST in controlled laboratory conditions. The bST produced by the bacteria is purified and then injected into cattle.* [12]

A rather interesting aspect of recombinant DNA, which bST production is a part, is that *Escherichia coli*, an intestinal tract bacterium in animals and humans, is played around with and then injected back into dairy cows. This leads to a question about what role, if any, does this process play in the plethora of meat contamination recalls in recent years, especially since slaughterhouses are steeped in animal feces.

Here's another case in point: the non-steroidal anti-inflammatory animal drug *flunixin.* [13]

Nature and the natural process of evolution did not include recent chemical, biological, technological, and genetic modification interventions. These impact organisms at various levels of their existence and reproductive cycles in recent times. Consider 'smart dust' [14] in chemtrails—those crisscross contrail-like patterns deliberately sprayed by U.S. military airplanes that expand into blanket-like clouds to enhance the U.S. government's HAARP [15] apparent weather control program. What chemicals do they contribute to the food chain? Aluminum, arsenic, barium, and boron per laboratory test results [16] are confirmed as being sprayed along with other agents.

Certainly such man-made chemistry was not a part of the evolutionary food chain humans have evolved with over thousands of years. Particularly disturbing to all life forms' DNA are fission-created nuclear radioactive isotopes released from nuclear power plants that impregnate foods growing in the fields.

When radiation is released with gas, as it was at the Japanese reactors, the particles are carried by prevailing winds, and some will settle on the earth. Rain will knock more of the suspended particles to the ground. "There is an extremely complex interaction between the type of radionuclide and the weather and the type of vegetation," Dr. Whicker said. "There can be hot spots far away from an accident, and places in between that are fine."

The principal elements that have been released from reactors at the Fukushima Daiichi plant are iodine 131 and cesium 137. Cesium is dangerous because it is long-lived and travels easily through the food chain, continuing to emit particles for centuries once it is released.

More than 15 years after the Chernobyl accident in what is now Ukraine, studies found that cesium 137 was still detectable in wild boar in Croatia and reindeer in Norway, with the levels high enough in some areas to pose a potential danger to people who consume a great deal of the meat.

While iodine 131 is much shorter lived — its radioactive potency is halved every eight days — it is dangerous because it concentrates in the thyroid gland, resulting in high radiation doses to that vulnerable organ. The thyroid is such an iodine magnet that Dr. Whicker recounts that a week after a nuclear weapons test in China, iodine 131 could be detected in the thyroid glands of deer in Colorado, although it could not be detected in the air or in nearby vegetation.

Initially, some plants will collect more radiation than others: those with big leaves like lettuce, spinach and other greens will naturally collect more radiation than apples, oranges or potatoes, he said. Foods like rice and corn whose edible portion is protected by husks or leaves are relatively safe in this early stage. [17]

And yet, no government health agency has issued health warnings about that. Therein may be the crux to global health problems: *mis-*information, *suppressed* information, or 'politically correct' Big Agra food industry data that government agencies and the medical professions propagate as healthful and health-enhancing information.

Here are just two examples of such food fallacies:

Trans fats [margarine in particular] which MDs and dietitians promoted as 'heart healthy foods' since the 1950s, whereas in reality they damage the entire cardiovascular system. The damage trans fats do to the body recently has been recognized and there even are laws prohibiting trans fats in restaurant foods. This is what the Mayo Clinic says about trans fats:

> *Trans fat is double trouble for your heart health. Trans fat raises your "bad" (LDL) cholesterol and lowers your "good" (HDL). Find out more about trans fat and how to avoid it.* [18]

Sugar is a health danger, especially high fructose corn syrup that food processors are desperately trying to eliminate from their products because of the implications it has for contributing to obesity. Sugar is ubiquitous and a staple in most processed foods. A former FDA administrator says this about sugar:

> *What we have to keep in mind,* says Walter Glinsmann, the FDA administrator who was the primary author of the 1986 report and who now is an adviser to the Corn Refiners Association, *is that sugar and high-fructose corn syrup might be toxic, as Lustig argues, but so might any substance if it's consumed in ways or in quantities that are unnatural for humans.* [19]

Did you catch Glinsmann's key phrase—"*unnatural for humans*"? Man-made food chemicals—usually from the petro-chemical industry—certainly are unnatural for humans, I think.

Regarding sugar, have you heard that sugar feeds cancer cells? Well, that probably is a secret food processors and others don't want you to know, since some form of sugar—cane, beet, corn fructose, etc.—is in most commercially produced edibles.

Tumor cells thrive on sugar, but they use fructose to pro-liferate. [20] "Importantly, fructose and glucose metabolism are quite different," Heaney's team wrote. …U.S. consumption of high fructose corn syrup went up 1,000 percent between 1970 and 1990, researchers reported in 2004 in the *American Journal of Clinical Nutrition.*

Note: The unaltered or crude cancer death rate per 100,000 U.S. populations for the year 1970 was162.8. …Twenty years later, the unaltered cancer death rate for the year 1990 …rose to 203.2. [21]

According to Nobel Prize recipient Dr Otto Warburg,

> *"Cancer has only one prime cause. It is the replacement of normal oxygen respiration of the body's cells by an anaerobic [i.e., oxygen-deficient] cell respiration."* ...
>
> But what else does Warburg's discovery tell us. First off, it tells us that cancer metabolizes much differently than normal cells. Normal cells need oxygen. Cancer cells despise oxygen. In fact, oxygen therapy is a favorite among many of the alternative clinics we've researched.
>
> **Another thing this tells us is that cancer metabolizes through a process of fermentation.** [22] [CJF emphasis added]

If you've ever made wine, you'll know that fermentation requires sugar.

All that fermentation produces yeast or a fungal microorganism known as *candida* in the body, which plays havoc and encourages cancer cell growth. Most 8 ounces of soda contain 7 teaspoons of sugar, more than a candy bar. And yet, the public is not told these unhealthful nutritional facts about sugars that impact our health and the etiology and growth of cancerous tumors.

As a trained *natural* nutritionist, I could cite several more examples, but I think you get where I'm going. I think consumers cannot trust the spin on nutrition put out by Big Agra and the food processing industry, which uses hundreds of thousands of pounds of additives, preservatives, and other food processing chemicals that add to the toxic burdens of our health and lives, plus most likely influence the growth of tumors in the body.

If you want to know how many food additives there are, please consider studying the U.S. Food and Drug Administration's "Food Additives Status List" [23]. Maybe you ought to be prepared to spend an entire day reading it.

Some claim

> *The annual production of bread alone is estimated to involve the addition of 10000000 pounds of chemical emulsifiers by thousands of bakers ... preservatives, flavouring and colouring matter, and a legion of processing agents.* [24]

That's ten *MILLION* pounds of chemicals in commercially produced bread alone.

In my last book, *Our Chemical Lives And The Hijacking Of Our DNA, A Probe Into What's Probably Making Us Sick,* [25] I discuss food and other DNA-altering chemical issues in greater detail, including copious peer-review and government research, data, and documentation.

Food, basically, has become a "Trojan horse" of sorts. All sorts of chemicals, neurotoxins, and poisons either are grown—now with genetically modified foods (GE or GMOs)—or manufactured/processed within it, as with nanoparticles. Such aggressive and dynamic food chemistry was heretofore unknown and foreign to human body chemistry. It places another dimension of biochemical involvement on the original intent of food that over evolutionary time evolved to include vitamins, minerals, trace minerals, amino acids, enzymes, metalloenzymes, antioxidants, carbohydrates, protein, fats and essential fatty acids, fiber, flavonoids, and yet-to-be-identified nutrients—without those synthetic, toxic, and chemical additives, plus transgenic DNA tinkering.

There's an old Yiddish idiom that says, "Health begins in the pot." Nothing can be more factual. However, the manner in which one prepares food plays a vital role in conserving and/or destroying nutrients and nutritional values. Frying and charbroiling food create carcinogenic particulates and polycyclic aromatic hydrocarbons (PACs). When I studied nutrition, I learned that a quarter-pound hamburger broiled/cooked over an open fire/flame had as many PAC carcinogenic particulates as did the smoke of 600 cigarettes.

Recently we learned about 'pink slime' or ammoniated beef trimmings in ground hamburger meat. We have to question what that may add to the PAC equation.

Food must be taken seriously as humans' primary health modality, especially when dealing with cancer. As Hippocrates, the Father of Medicine, is quoted as saying, *"Let food be thy medicine and medicine be thy food."*

The current state of nutrient content and educational campaigns by food processors leave a lot to be desired, in my opinion. There is too much technological intervention in growing and processing food crops—from fertilizers to pesticides to genetically modified seeds and organisms (Transgenic and Cisgenic) to additives and preservatives—that destroy or prevent nutrient rich foods from being consumed. One testimonial to that is the rate of obesity for both children and adults, particularly in the United States. In the USA there are 58 million people overweight; 40 million obese, 3 million morbidly obese, and 8 out of 10 people over 25 years of age are overweight. That's one-third of the population with weight problems. Obesity is the number 2 cause of preventable death in the USA. Obesity also can be a contributing factor in some cancers.

If you look at old films and newsreels from the 1940s and 1950s, you never see humans like 'waddle ducks' on streets and in public places. Another lifestyle convenience you never see in those films is the ubiquitous fast food restaurant chains. As a nation, we were much healthier then as the food chemistry industry had not yet taken over, and cancer was virtually unknown. I know of medical doctors who were in med school then whose entire classes were called to a cancer patient's room, as cancers were a rarity back then. My, how things have changed!

Fat doesn't mean well fed; it means the opposite: undernourished and overfed on sugar, high starch carbohydrates, and processed grains, snacks, sodas, and edibles that convert into fat within the body.

Organically grown foods usually offer rich nutrients from sustainable agriculture food sources, i.e., fruits, vegetables, grains, dairy, and animal meats/products. Organically grown foods provide the best possible nutrient-dense foods you can purchase and eat, depending upon how little you process them. If you cook the enzymes out of fresh raw vegetables, they become less nutritious. Raw food enzymes are the key to health. The *Gerson Therapy* for managing cancers is based in raw food enzymes and juicing.

For years we have heard that cabbage family vegetables— *Brassicaceae*—are important anti-cancer foods. I highly recommend them in various sections of this book where I talk about diet and nutrition because those vegetables contain *di-indolmethane* [DIM], which can be an excellent estrogen controller for cancers of *the breast, uterus, prostate and other reproductive tissue.*

> *DIM has been shown to help regulate and promote a more efficient metabolism of estrogen, and an optimal ratio of estrogen metabolites. DIM is thought to be responsible for the health effects of dietary Indole-3-Carbinol (I3C).* [26]

The following information is of particular importance in understanding why Indole-3-Carbinol (I3C) needs to become a HUGE percentage of your *daily diet* in managing breast cancer. I cannot agree more with this observation:

> *Research since the 1970s has determined that disrupted estrogen metabolism is closely linked to several health risks in men and women, particularly those involving the breast, uterus, prostate and other reproductive tissue. Genetics, excess weight, poor diet and other lifestyle factors may result in an imbalance of estrogen metabolites.* **Xenoestrogenic**

***compounds of the modern world, such as organo-
chlorine pesticides, can significantly disrupt healthy
estrogen metabolism.*** [CJF emphasis added] [26]

That highlighted sentence is extremely important in understanding the urgency and need to remove *all* pesticides, herbicides, insecticides, rodenticides, 'camphor balls', etc. from your
environment at home, work, and the food you eat. Many pesticide chemicals act as endocrine disruptors or "hormone copy-
cats," particularly imitating female hormones, which also—and
definitely—affect the male prostate and PSA test values.

I know I had exposure to chemical fumes and vapors—a
next-door neighbor used to spray herbicides very frequently.
That also probably contributed to what happened to me, as
I've lived a holistic life-style since I was in my early thirties.
Petrochemicals really do a number on the human body sooner
or later. And yet our modern lifestyles are entrenched in them.
Think how often you spray for bugs; flea dip your pets; use weed
killers; light scented candles; use dryer sheets that impregnate
chemicals into clothes and bed linens—just take a whiff outside the dryer vent; eat untold quantities of additives, preservatives, and food processing chemicals *daily* without knowing
how they interact within the body, since chemical interaction
testing has not been done either by government health agencies
nor those chemical companies who manufacture them.

*The phytochemicals in cruciferous vegetables have been shown
to beneficially affect the body's hormonal and detoxification*

systems. **Epidemiological studies have supported the health benefits of consuming these vegetables.** [26] [CJF emphasis added]

In my last book, *Our Chemical Lives And The Hijacking Of Our DNA*, I devote Chapter 9 to *Endocrine Disruptors—Not My Pesticides?*

Additional Information

To understand the connection between healthy soil and healthy-healthful food, you may want to listen to Jeff Moyer, Farm Manager, Rodale Institute and former chair of the National Organic Standards Board, who discusses organic agriculture, the science behind it, non-chemically grown foods, and biological systems. He was a guest on KOPN.FM August 18, 2011. [27] You may access that program online at <kopn.org/aasp?u=http://kopn.org/a/showrss4.php?n=http://kopn.org/dc/dircaster2.php?p=fs>.

After reading this chapter I hope you can get some idea as to what's going on biochemically within the human body today; the reasons so many people 'enjoy' such poor health; and the need to revise attitudes and approaches to food and eating for managing breast cancer.

Don't let your worries get the better of you; 'cause all you need to do is remember that Moses started out life as a 'basket case'.

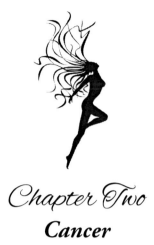

Chapter Two
Cancer

Cancer is a word, not a sentence.

… John Diamond

My cancer scare changed my life. I'm grateful for every new, healthy day I have. It has helped me prioritize my life.

… *Olivia Newton-John*

*I*n some respects cancer has become a disease feared almost as leprosy (Hansen's disease) was feared in biblical times, except with one humongous difference: ***Cancer is a moneymaker*** for so many ancillary medical and health-related industries, professionals, and research, in particular.

There's no doubt that cancer has been occurring in humans in prior times, but the prevalence with which it's occurring in the last thirty to forty years is documented as increasing dramatically, and is outrageously unjustifiable, I think. People suffer with cancer mostly because of the chemicalized lifestyles that have been forced upon us as part of a modern society.

During World War I (1914-18) many chemicals were invented as war faring agents that were designed to kill the enemy. Mustard gas, tear gas (ethyl bromoacetate), phosgene, and chlorine came out of World War I chemical war technology.

> *The first killing agent employed by the German military was chlorine. German chemical companies BASF, Hoechst and Bayer (which formed the IG Farben conglomerate in 1925) had been producing chlorine as a by-product of their dye manufacturing.* [28]

Many of the above-mentioned chemical companies after the war became pharmaceutical companies.

Currently the chemical industry impacts every segment of business and society. Nothing says that more accurately than this information from the U.S. Department of Labor's website [29]

> *Chemical manufacturing is divided into seven segments, six of which are... basic chemicals, synthetic materials, agricultural chemicals, paint, coatings, and adhesives, cleaning preparations, and other chemical products. The seventh segment, pharmaceutical and medicine manufacturing,* which probably has the most impact of all on our lives.
> *The **basic chemicals segment** produces various petrochemicals, gases, dyes, and pigments. Petrochemicals*

contain carbon and hydrogen and are made primarily from petroleum and natural gas. The production of both organic and inorganic chemicals occurs in this segment. Organic chemicals are used to make a wide range of products, such as dyes, plastics, and pharmaceutical products; however, the majority of these chemicals are used in the production of other chemicals. Industrial inorganic chemicals usually are made from salts, metal compounds, other minerals, and the atmosphere. In addition to producing solid and liquid chemicals, firms involved in inorganic chemical manufacturing produce industrial gases such as oxygen, nitrogen, and helium. Many inorganic chemicals serve as processing ingredients in the manufacture of chemicals, but do not appear in the final products because they are used as catalysts—chemicals that speed up or otherwise aid a reaction.

The **synthetic materials segment** produces a wide variety of finished products as well as raw materials, including common plastic materials such as polyethylene, polypropylene, polyvinyl chloride (PVC), and polystyrene. Among products into which these plastics can be made are loudspeakers, toys, PVC pipes, and beverage bottles. This industry segment also produces plastic materials used for mixing and blending resins on a custom basis. Motor vehicle manufacturers are particularly large users of synthetic materials.

The **agricultural chemicals segment**, which employs the fewest workers in the chemical industry, supplies farmers and home gardeners with fertilizers, herbicides, pesticides, *and other agricultural chemicals. The segment also includes companies involved in the formulation and preparation of agricultural and household pest control chemicals.*

*The **paint, coating, and adhesive products segment** includes firms making paints, varnishes, putties, paint removers, sealers, adhesives, glues, and caulking. The construction and furniture industries are large customers of this segment. Other customers range from individuals refurbishing their homes to businesses needing anticorrosive paints that can withstand high temperatures.*

*The **cleaning preparations segment** is the only segment in which much of the production is geared directly toward consumers. The segment includes firms making soaps, detergents, and cleaning preparations. Cosmetics and toiletries, including perfume, lotion, and toothpaste, also are produced in this segment. Households and businesses use these products in many ways, cleaning everything from babies to bridges.*

*The **"other chemical" products segment** includes manufacturers of explosives, printing ink, film, toners, matches, and other miscellaneous chemicals. These products are used by consumers or in the manufacture of other products.*

***Recent developments. Nanotechnology** will continue to benefit all of the manufacturing industries. The advantages of the applications of nanotechnology have far from reached their limits, but research and development in nanotechnology are both expensive and time consuming.*

In the chemical manufacturing industry, developments in Nanotechnology will help conserve energy needed to produce chemicals and reduce the amount of waste products, making the manufacturing process more efficient. [CJF emphasis added]

Nanotechnology, now being implemented, probably may be the scariest of all since we really won't know what chemicals or other agents will be inserted into those micro-mini Trojan horses that will impact our lives, including information chips to be inserted under people's skin.

According to a September 2011 report in *The Lancet* [30] the number of new breast cancer cases rose dramatically between 1980 and 2010. In thirty years the number of breast cancers reported globally went from 641,000 to 1.6 MILLION. That's almost two-and-a-half times what it was just thirty years ago! Researchers theorized the increase was due to an aging female population, as older women are more vulnerable to contracting breast cancer.

Jan Coebergh, a cancer expert from Erasmus University Medical Centre in Rotterdam, the Netherlands, said of the study, *"People may wonder what the urgency is in addressing these cancers, but the numbers are staggering. It's like six jumbo jets crashing every day."*

According to the National Breast Cancer Coalition *Facts and Statistics about Breast Cancer in the United States – 2011,*

All women are at risk for breast cancer. Only 5-10% of those with breast cancer have inherited a mutation in the known breast cancer genes (BRCA1 and BRCA2) and 90-95% of breast cancer cases do not involve these inherited mutations. (ACS 2010; NCI 2006).

Factors that increase a woman's risk of breast cancer include older age, genetic factors, family history of breast or ovarian cancer, long menstrual history, null parity (having no children), older than 30 years of age at first full-term pregnancy, daily alcohol consumption, use of combined postmenopausal hormone replacement therapy (HRT), postmenopausal obesity and ionizing radiation. Factors that decrease a woman's risk of breast cancer include breastfeeding and physical activity (exercise) (ACS, 2010).

Studies on chemo preventive agents tamoxifen and raloxifene were not adequately designed to determine their impact on the prevention of breast cancer for healthy women, nor are the studies long enough to assess long term side effects and impact on mortality (Vogel et al, 2010). [31]

Something that needs to be highlighted appears in the second item: ionizing radiation as a factor that increases a woman's risk of breast cancer. So why does allopathic medicine use mammograms, which produce ionizing radiation, as a diagnostic tool or procedure? Good question? See Chapter 9, *Radiation, What Is It?* for more about it.

Equally ironic, I think, is nowhere do we see chemicals as a cause of cancer or as a gene-modifying factor, and yet numerous animal studies indicate just how many cancers are caused by them. I discuss that in great depth in my book *Our*

Chemical Lives And The Hijacking Of Our DNA available on Amazon.com. A possible clue as to why chemicals are not mentioned, I think, is in the third item where we find talk about chemo preventive drugs, the basis upon which the allopathic medical paradigm is based: pharmaceuticals, which are man-made *patented* chemicals. There's a clue.

Stepping aside for a moment and not discriminating against toxic chemicals, but talking about metals that also cause DNA mutations and cancer, I'd like to share the story about toothpaste tubes that were made of lead—yes lead—and aluminum. It wasn't until the 1970s that plastic was used to make toothpaste tubes. Can you imagine what a load of toxic metals probably was brushed into the very absorbent tissues of the buccal cavity—the mouth—from using toothpaste dispensed in lead and aluminum tubes?

Toothpaste in a tube was the brainchild of Dr Washington Sheffield in 1892, after years of his selling *Sheffield's Crème Dentrifice* in jars. The entriguing story about toothpaste tubes appears in Shelley Moore's article "About Toothpaste Tubes Made of Metal." [32]

To learn more about toxic metals and the roles they play in disease(s), you may want to read Chapter 19 *Toxic and Heavy Metals* in my book, *Our Chemical Lives And The Hijacking Of Our DNA, A Probe Into What's Probably Making Us Sick.*

However the book you are reading now seriously deals with breast cancer by *not putting* more *toxic* chemicals and *toxic* metals into a body that already is biochemically compromised. An important aspect, I think and used, was to go on four detoxification programs that over the course of several months extracted as many chemicals as my body would give up by activating my lymphatic and immune systems. I did that using a liquid homeopathic program from Italy, *Guna Biotherapeutics Detox Treatment.* [33]

I chose that holistic protocol *instead* of putting more chemicals into my body that probably would make me horrendously sick, lose my hair, and possibly give me a secondary cancer. Incidentally, those side effects have been the unfortunate documented history of chemotherapy—and knowing that—was the second-most important reason for my choosing the holistic route. My side effects were pimples breaking out on my face, back, and arms that once they opened and released the toxins, healed and my skin was clear again. The first comment people make about me is, "Look at your skin! Its' unbelievably beautiful for your age."

Never borrow from the future because if you worry about what may happen tomorrow and it doesn't, you then have worried in vain. However, if it does happen, you will have worried twice. That's not healthy.

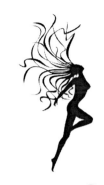

Chapter Three
Breast Physiology

*All truths are easy to understand once they are discovered;
the point is to discover them.*

... Galileo Galilei (1564—1642)
**Italian astronomer persecuted by the
church for saying the sun was the center of the universe**

To understand female breast physiology we need to go back as far as *female in utero development,* i.e., during the nine months of gestation and pregnancy in her mother's womb.

At 7 to 8 weeks *in utero*, the first stages of mammary development begin.

During the third trimester (7th thru 9th months of gestation) placental hormones induce breast duct formation.

Between the 32nd to 40th weeks *in utero*, lactation breast lobules develop.

However, when a female becomes pregnant, another series of breast events take place:

During the first trimester [first 3 months of pregnancy] breast enlargement takes place from ductal sprouting due to the predominance of the female hormone estrogen.

During the second trimester [4th thru 6th months of pregnancy] progesterone takes precedence and is responsible for breast maturation and lobule differentiation.

Birthing the child activates prolactin for milk production, which provides immune factors for the newborn infant.

And there's another time in a female's life when breast tissue gets impacted, that is post-menopausal.

Basically, stroma tissue shrinks leaving more fatty tissue. Stroma is connective tissue that supports milk ducts and glands. When it shrinks, that's the start of women's breasts "going south," losing their 'perkiness', and also when cells can experience gene mutations. Mutations can occur in either the epithelium where milk ducts and glands are located—the more usual site of cell and gene changes—or in the stroma, which is thought to be a more uncommon site for cell mutation and more difficult to detect. Women with dense stromal breast tissue are more prone to gene mutations. Furthermore, high-density connective tissue seems more likely to experience gene mutations.

Not all breast tumors are cancerous and here's a list to relieve your mind.

Fibroadenomas are benign breast tumors that commonly appear in women under 35 years of age.

Phyllode tumors have epithelial cells that are benign, but stromal tissue is malignant.

Harmatoma of the breast usually is a benign tumor composed of connective tissue, fat, and glandular tissue occurring in females over 35 years of age.

Vascular tumors are benign and usually less than 2 centimeters in size, localized with no growth infiltration.

Granular cell tumors are benign but upon palpation are rock hard and simulate a cancerous tumor.

Stromal tumors can be either lipomas [fat containing tumors] or liposacromas, which are rare, but are cancerous components within phyllode tumors.

Fibrocystic Breast Change is benign and due to hormonal changes in the female body. It involves lobes, glandular ducts, and connective breast tissue most common in females between the ages of 20 and 50. Fibrocystic changes can be felt in one or both breasts and are regulated by the menstrual cycle. Most females experience some sort of fibrocystic change during their lifetime. However, if a cyst seems hard, please get it checked out by your physician. Cysts do show up on ultrasound examinations, if you are concerned about mammography. Caffeine, chocolate, and cola-type sodas have impact upon fibrocystic swelling and breast pain. It would be a good practice to omit them from your eating plan even if you don't experience fibrocystic changes, especially if you are at an age when post menopausal breast changes will start to occur.

Between 1975 and 1987 there was a precipitous rise in female breast cancer rates in the United States. That also coincided with the exorbitant rise in chemicals used in food growing and processing, along with escalation of the fast food restaurant phenomenon.

Stanford University in California has been doing research into finding ways to turn off cancer cells, i.e., shut down the genes that cause cancer. There are numerous *natural plant* agents women have been using for years that do just that. However, these natural plant biological elements cannot be patented and big pharma can't make mega bucks from them. Perhaps research scientists will keep on searching until they can come up with an ingredient they can patent into a pharmaceutical for big pharma, who can charge megabucks for them so health insurance providers can be billed. It's all about corporate profits, it seems, otherwise many *effective* cancer-fighting plants would have been mainstreamed into allopathic cancer treatments long ago.

A significant tell tale factor regarding female breast cancer, I think, can be found in the fact that it is highest in developed countries with western lifestyles such as the USA, Canada, Northern Europe, Australia, and New Zealand. Interestingly, the lowest rates of female breast cancer are found in African and Asian countries, where more people grow their own food, live off and closer to the land.

Epidemiological studies found that Asian-American women born in the USA had higher breast cancer risk/rate percentages than Asian-American women born in Asia. Also, after Asian women immigrants have lived in the USA for many years, they developed a significant higher risk for breast cancer as compared with recent Asian immigrant women.

An Unrecognized Form of Breast Cancer
Inflammatory Breast Cancer (IBC)

Breast cancer most often is considered in terms of tumors or a mass in the breast. Even though they may be the predominant symptoms and diagnoses, there is another form that often defies detection by both patient and her physician; it's inflammatory breast cancer, the symptoms of which need to be recognized for what they indicate. Since many general practitioners often miss inflammatory breast cancer symptoms, my suggestion is to go to a women's health clinic where they are more experienced in diagnosing IBC.

Inflammatory breast cancer symptoms often are regarded as anything from an insect bite to a rash to an inflamed nerve ending to an ordinary infection to just about anything *except* cancer. Itching and/or a stinging/burning sensation in the breast need immediate medical diagnostic attention, as does any symptom that presents on or within the breast. Redness, swelling, and an unusual configuration of the breast nipple, usually resembling an inversion, must get immediate attention. Swollen lymph node(s) under an armpit is definitely another symptom.

As an aside, I'd like to caution women about using antiperspirants and deodorants that contain aluminum and other harsh chemicals, especially after shaving underarms. Toxins and chemicals can migrate into the lymph nodes. Skin tissue is permeable; think of medical patches with medication in them.

An effective way to deal with underarm perspiration is to keep them shaved and each morning swab them with a cotton ball saturated with hydrogen peroxide. It seems heavy-duty meat eaters tend to have odorous underarm perspiration.

IBC is an aggressive form of cancer that blocks lymph vessels. Even though it is considered rare, it causes somewhere between one and five percent of all female breast cancers. Often physicians *do not* recognize its symptoms. The reason it is called inflammatory breast cancer is because the breast most often is red, swollen, or inflamed. Women must know that mammograms are not effective in detecting IBC.

The most effective diagnostic procedure for IBC is Thermography—see Chapter 45—which registers the amount of heat coming off an inflamed breast and converts it into a photographic assay. Cancer cells emit heat, which thermography 'sees' and captures, whereas mammograms can't register IBC as they only 'see' tumors or masses within breast tissue that are large enough to be detected.

There is an educational video about IBC that is helpful in understanding a form of breast cancer most women either never heard of or physicians honestly—and regrettably—don't recognize. May I suggest your visiting the Internet website *Health Watch's* <youtube.com/watch?v=mmKWHvDy0yM&feature=player_embedded>.

For more information about IBC, you may want to access Internet sites such as:
- Inflammatory Breast Cancer Research Foundation at <ibcresearch.org/>.
- Inflammatory Breast Cancer Association Definition, Signs and Symptoms at <ibchelp.org>.

- IBC Support: Inflammatory Breast Cancer Help and Support at <ibcsupport.org/>.

Laugh! And then laugh some more. It's good for you.

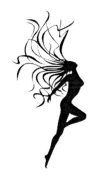

Chapter Four
MALE Breast Cancer

The mass of men lead lives of quiet desperation.

… Henry David Thoreau (1817—1862)
Author, *Walden*

reast cancer can—and does—occur in men. Statistically, breast cancer in men is only one percent of all breast cancers with about two thousand new cases diagnosed each year. Most male breast cancers develop in men between 50 and 60 years of age.

According to the Mayo Clinic, that facility provides basically the same diagnostics for males as females: digital mammography, magnetic resonance imaging (MRI), ultrasound, stereotactic breast biopsies, MRI-guided breast biopsies and surgical biopsies. Furthermore, postoperative treatment can include radiation and chemotherapy. [34]

Some men joke about having *"male boobs,"* which basically have similar tissue to female breasts—including milk glands—but more *under-developed* than female breast tissue.

Interestingly, exposure to ionizing radiation is associated with developing breast cancer in males. Mammography produces ionizing radiation.

High levels of the female hormone estrogen are considered the true cause for male breast cancer. I'd also like to add chemical exposure. Drinking beer and other alcoholic beverages could alter the levels of hormones in the blood, thereby increasing female hormones in males. That may be something to consider. *Gynecomastia* is the medical term for male breast enlargement due to an elevated level of the female hormone estrogen. Some prescription medications also can induce gynecomastia.

According to *Medscape,*[35] these drugs can induce gynecomastia:

> *Estrogens or drugs with estrogenlike activity - Include diethylstilbestrol, digitalis, and phytoestrogens, as well as estrogen-contaminated food and estrogen-containing cosmetics*
>
> *Drugs that enhance estrogen synthesis - Include gonadotropins, clomiphene, phenytoin, and exogenous testosterone*
>
> *Drugs that inhibit testosterone synthesis or action - Include ketoconazole, metronidazole, alkylating agents, cisplatin, spironolactone, cimetidine, flutamide, finasteride, and etomidate*
>
> *Drugs that act by unknown mechanisms - Include isonicotinic acid hydrazide, methyldopa, busulfan, tricyclic antidepressants, diazepam, penicillamine, omeprazole,*

phenothiazines, calcium channel blockers, angiotensin-converting enzyme (ACE) inhibitors, alcohol, marijuana, and heroin

For those who love munchies and junk food snacks, I'd like to remind you they often are filled with MSG—monosodium glutamate, which is an excitotoxin that produces free radicals in body tissue capable of causing cancer. You may want to keep in mind that constant exposure to free radicals can promote oncogenes and tumor growth. Maybe knocking off the Saturday night six-pack, pretzels, chips, and junk food could be a preventive health measure in addition to losing weight and a beer belly.

Male breast cancer patients also can utilize information in this book about holistic female breast cancer treatments. To learn what allopathic medicine has to say about male breast cancer, you may want to visit the American Cancer Society's website *Breast Cancer in Men* at <cancer.org/Cancer/BreastCancerinMen/DetailedGuide/breast-cancer-in-men-what-is-breast-cancer-in-men>.

Not to digress from the main topic of this book, female breast cancer, but I'd like my readers to know about some very exciting news regarding *male prostate cancer* that broke while I was writing this book. Australian researchers found a way to starve prostate cancer cells.

Researchers at the Centenary Institute in Sydney have discovered a potential future treatment for prostate cancer – through starving the tumour [sic] *cells of an essential nutrient they need to grow rapidly. Their work, with human cells grown in the lab, reveals targets for drugs that could slow the progress of early and late stage prostate cancer.*

Current therapies for prostate cancer include surgical removal of the prostate, radiation, freezing the tumour [sic] *or cutting off the supply of the hormone testosterone – but there are often side-effects including incontinence and impotence.*

Growing cells need an essential nutrient, the amino acid called leucine, which is pumped into the cell by specialised [sic] *proteins. And this could be prostate cancer's weak link.* Reference: *Science Daily,* Nov. 2, 2011

This *starving of cancer cells* is what holistic cancer treatments are all about and that's what I've been doing in my program with my specialized diet, multiple and mega-nutrients, and specific holistic therapies like vitamin C intravenous drips weekly *instead* of pharmaceutical chemotherapies.

However, what would you like to wager that Australian researchers are looking for a chemical drug that can be patented to starve cancer cells to death and make megabucks for Big Pharma? That's probably what it's all about, not curing cancer, which can be and is being done using holistic therapies. What I'd like my readers to know is that you can do it right now with a special and strict diet, nutritional supplements, and other natural therapies that starve cancer cells. I know; I'm doing it, and it's working.

Don't think too much; you may weaken the team.

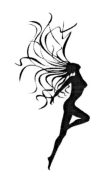

Chapter Five

The 'Psycho-Bio-Physiological Chemistry' That Surrounds Cancer

Attitude is a little thing that makes a big difference.

**… Sir Winston Churchill (1874—1965)
British Prime Minister/Statesman**

One of the least apparent, yet more prominent, aspects in cancer management is the role that head games play—some often brought on by medical spin, physicians, surgeons, or healthcare professionals—that can be quite intimidating, if not upsetting. Early on I realized just how vituperative some really could be and, especially, from sources one would least expect. From my experience, I can only imagine what many women must go through.

Trying to get one's head around dealing with breast cancer is frightening and challenging enough, but having to deal with angst supplied by doctors, family, and friends who think you should take treatment for breast cancer their way, truly is most upsetting.

As a consumer healthcare researcher I knew—and know—more about the politics of cancer—and healthcare issues in general—than most consumers do, so I decided a very long time ago that if I ever were confronted with a cancer scare, I would manage it via non-toxic methods and not subject my body to the accepted route of surgery-radiation-chemotherapy, often dubbed the "cut, burn, and poison cure." My treatment decision literally blew some folks' minds when I shared it with them.

Of course I had opposition from the medical profession when I said I didn't want a mammogram; instead, I opted for thermography and a sonogram. After the sonogram, I was pressured to take a mammogram that would subject my breasts to possible damage from ionizing radiation, plus a possibility of breaking open the two tumors and spreading cells from the pressure of 55 to 60 pounds of weight from mammogram plates squashing my breast. Any female who has had a mammogram knows how painful the procedure really is on sensitive mammary glands—the female breasts.

> *Because there is no safe dose (risk-free dose) of ionizing radiation, we can be certain at the outset that mammographic programs will cause some number of radiation-induced breast-cancers. The question is: How many?* [36]

So why would I subject my breasts to a procedure that could most likely be a cancer-causing diagnostic procedure when I already had a confirming thermogram and sonogram? I politely dismissed the radiologist.

There is something, though, that has always concerned me about mammograms ever since I can remember: They can cause cancer, as the above quote indicates, so why use a diagnostic procedure that is known to induce cancer? That just doesn't make sense, when there is a perfectly reliable and *FDA-approved diagnostic* available that even is more accurate than mammograms—even at very early stages of cancer cell growth, even before a mammogram is capable of detecting a tumor. Thermography does not shoot ionizing radiation into the breast and body. I'll talk more about that in chapters 9, 11, 12, and 45.

Kaiser Health News published an interview with Dr Barron Lerner about **the politics of mammography and breast cancer,** part of which I'd like to quote because it demonstrates what's really the issue I think, not women's health, but politics:

> *Q: Congress has legislated about breast cancer in the past – can you tell us about that?*
>
> *A: In the late 1990s, Congress passed a bill that mandated that women who had a mastectomy would have their reconstructive surgery paid for. If you think about this, this really doesn't happen in most areas except for breast cancer, where Congress would act, and say, "This is something we're forcing insurance companies to do."* **But it speaks to the powerful nature of the breast-cancer lobby. One other time a report came out criticizing mammograms,** *Congress actually voted – I think the House voted 430 to nothing [ed. note: it was 424-0] – to rebuke that*

scientific report. **So, politics is always intruding into the world of breast cancer.** [37] [CJF emphasis added]

Would you like read that last sentence again and let it sink in?

Therein lies the problem with breast cancer treatments, and medicine in general: Powerful lobbying groups with very deep pockets whose contents (megabucks) are very influential with Congress and the FDA, in particular. Maureen Glabman says,

The "right ... to petition the government" has come a long way in over 200 years, and health care organizations are not shy in exercising it.

[There are] 17,800 registered Washington lobbyists upon whom interest groups spent $1.56 billion last year [2001] to sway Congress and the executive branch — numbers that are grossly understated due to the narrow definition of "registered lobbyist," says Jeffrey Birnbaum, author of The Lobbyists: How Influence Peddlers Get Their Way in Washington.

An estimated 40 percent of those 17,800 lobbyists promote health care agendas, according to James Albertine, president of the Alexandria, Va.-based American League of Lobbyists. To put it another way, there are 13 health care lobbyists for each of the 535 members of Congress. Among their most passionate causes this year are Medicare reimbursements and tort reform.

Hundreds of medical groups have a lobbying presence in Washington. The AMA — the third-largest lobbying

group (based on expenditures) — spent about $17 million in 2000, the latest year for which figures are available.

What often goes unrecognized, however, is that while lobbyists bring home legislative gifts to hungry member-ships, they also aid members of Congress in drafting com-plex medical legislation. [38]

Here's an example of some lobbying groups budgets for the year 2000. One can only imagine what their current [2012] lobbying budgets are.

Sampling of medical lobbyist budgets in 2000

Blue Cross Blue Shield Association	$8.0 million
American Association of Health Plans	$3.6 million
American College of Physicians/ASIM	$2.1 million
American Academy of Family Physicians	$1.6 million

Source: Center for Responsive Politics

Of the **2006 top lobbyists**, the *American Hospital Association* ranked number 6 with a budget of $11.9 million. So, is there any wonder why women don't have a say about non-toxic treatment and management for breast cancer, when such influential financial lobbying interests have the power to keep non-toxic and effective cancer treatments out of main-stream healthcare practice, information, and health insurance coverage? The most common denigrate allopathic medicine presents about non-toxic treatments is that holistic treatments offer false hope by "quacks," which I'd like to challenge with the following rebuttal.

My rationale for challenging allopathic medicine's denigrate of holistic cancer treatments is this: Holistic medical doctors and professionals are state-licensed professionals who have realized that the 'cut-burn-poison' method of cancer treatment does more damage to the patient and, as responsible healthcare professionals, they want to give their patients *non-toxic and immune-enhancing* regimens, modalities, and protocols rather than toxic chemicals and treatments that often lead to secondary cancers years later. Many cancer patients now are agreeing with such a philosophy and are seeking treatments that are holistic and humane.

The Washington Post columnist Dan Eggen wrote an article [July 21, 2009] titled "Lobbyists Spend Millions to Influence Health Care" that seems to illustrate much of what is going on:

> *New disclosure reports that began arriving Monday in Congress showed familiar players at the top of the health-care influence heap, including $6.2 million in lobbying by the dominant Pharmaceutical Research and Manufacturers of America (PhRMA) and $4 million by the American Medical Association.*
>
> *Many health companies and associations increased their first-quarter lobbying expenditures, sometimes dramatically. The Blue Cross and Blue Shield Association upped its lobbying expenditures by a full million, to 2.8*

million dollars in the second quarter; GlaxoSmithKline's spending jumped from $1.8 million to $2.3 million; Novartis grew from $1.4 million to $1.8 million; and Metlife Group reported $1.7 million, up nearly 50 percent. Allstate, which spent less than $900,000 on lobbying through March, boosted its spending to more than $1.5 million from April to June. [39]

Lobbyists for the mammogram monopoly operate similarly. Consider this:

Alice Mundy of The Wall Street Journal reports: "The final health-care bill is likely to require coverage for more mammograms than the new guidelines recommend after women's groups, doctors and imaging-equipment makers stepped up pressure on lawmakers—one of many threads of the bill negotiated behind the scenes." [40]

General Electric and Siemens AG—both manufacture mammography equipment—are heavy donors to pro-mammogram advocacy groups, e.g., The American College of Radiology and *Susan G. Komen for the Cure.*

Bucking big *pro*-mammography bucks in support of non-toxic breast cancer screening and management certainly is right up there with other head games involved in breast cancer issues. It seems corporations with vested interests ply their wares in apparently best interests of themselves and their products, rather than patients, I think, because their actions leave no room for either professional competition or insurance reimbursement for non-toxic and totally effective diagnostic screening, modalities, and treatment. I think a *quid quo pro* exists between such corporations, Congress, and federal health agencies, plus the cancer industry also gets a "Get Out of Jail Free" card from Congress and government oversight agencies, since much of their propaganda is spin control to create fear and a need with a resulting automatic lock-step acceptance of toxic cancer treatments since President Nixon declared the "War on Cancer" in 1971—over forty years ago.

Therein lies a great part of the problem: *accepted media spin and advertising.* Just listen to all the radio ads for cancer hospital treatment centers—that terrifies healthcare consumers into accepting toxic therapies, which, in most instances, do not provide cures since most statistical reporting is being uncovered as skewed or downright false.

> *The false statistics trap can be quite damaging to the quest for knowledge. For example, in medical science, correcting a falsehood may take decades and cost lives.* [41]

Secondary cancers often are an unfortunate legacy for conventional allopathic breast cancer treatments.

Fear—a real head game—plays an integral part in cancer management, I think. Personally, I feel the medical profession probably is more afraid of cancer than patients, which only promotes more anxiety for cancer patients. Here's some information that may be just what you need to know regarding safe, effective, and non-toxic diagnostic procedures from Dr Lynn Morales, ND:

> *There are also tests that are actually better than mammograms. Simple blood tests, which are routinely administered **after a mastectomy** to determine if any cancer is still present, should be the screening test of choice **before any radical treatment**. The best of these are **tumor marker** tested called **Cancer Antigen 15-3 (CA 15-3)** and **Cancer Antigen 27-29 (CA 27-29)**. When your doctor prescribes repeated mammograms, just ask him or her for a tumor marker test. There are no cancer tests that are 100% accurate. But at least with this testing, procedure is non-invasive and a clear yes or no answer is provided. If you are in the high-risk group for whatever reason, you can have a CA 15-3 every 3-4 months. … [CJF emphasis added]*
>
> *And remember, when it comes to screening, proceed cautiously with mammograms, and be sure to use alternative, tumor market [sic] testing. Despite the uproar, the medical scientists who analyzed all the data and determined that we should use fewer mammograms deserve applause-they have done a great service to all women nationwide.* [42]

Perhaps this would be an appropriate place to tell women about the *Journal of the American Medical Association* article "Detection of Breast Cancer With Addition of Annual Screening Ultrasound or a Single Screening MRI to Mammography in

Women With Elevated Breast Cancer Risk," published April 4, 2012, wherein ultrasound alone caught an additional 32 percent breast cancers and MRI by itself uncovered an additional 8 percent. [43]

Games—games are played with women's lives inadvertently. Sometimes the *opposing team* isn't recognized until it becomes rather late in the game. Regardless, women should not permit vested interest spin control and games to get into our heads, thereby inducing fear and influencing our choices for treatment. That, of course, is what they want and will do everything possible to plant the 'fear of God' in breast cancer patients.

That and influencing the power of the purse—health insurance reimbursement policies deny some non-toxic diagnostics and most treatments, which keep conventional medicine's 'cut-burn-poison' treatments regarded as the 'gold standard'.

All the above probably amounts to or feels like psychological warfare that females—and some men—encounter when confronted with breast cancer issues. The negative effects such psychological issues generate within a cancer-compromised body and immune system certainly program and determine less than optimum biological and physiological chemistry pathways in a cancer patient. David Spiegel, MD, talks about the body and mind being one and calls it *"body-mind connection medicine"* that few healthcare practitioners, except holistic practitioners, take seriously and actually employ in their practice for cancer management, I think.

Having a positive outlook on one's ability to cope and heal, rather than living in constant fear and anxiety, allows for the release of endorphins, the body's natural healing agents. When our bodies stimulate endorphin production, studies have documented numerous benefits: pain reduction, a mollification of stress hormones—cortisol, in particular, that is produced by the adrenal glands, improved blood pressure management and readings, and most of all, enhancement of the immune system, which cancer patients really need.

That very subject is covered in the book *Heal Yourself: Using the Scientifically Proven Mind-Body Connection to Manage Chronic Pain, Depression, Cancer and More,* by Dr Lynne Zimmerman. The message Dr Zimmerman's book imparts is that you can change the chemical signals the brain sends to organs and every system in your body to effectuate healing and wellness.

Back in the 1970s Norman Cousins [1915-1990] healed himself of a life-threatening disease [*Anklyosing Spondylitis,* a collagen disease that attacks the connective tissues of the body] by watching funny movies and reading funny stories—literally laughing his illness into wellness. Subsequently, Cousins wrote a book about that experience, *Anatomy of an Illness,* which is available on Amazon.com, wherein he documents how laughter and feeling good about himself enabled him to get off painkiller and sleeping pills quickly with the additional benefit of sleeping better. Sleep is most important in healing the body, and anything that can enhance one's ability to get quality sleep certainly is most important. Worry, fear, anxiety, and adverse effects from chemotherapy or radiation—coupled with nausea and other side effects—certainly interfere with many patients and their ability to sleep.

Anyone who has an illness—and cancer patients, in particular—needs to understand that attitude plays a major role in overcoming or managing a disease. There's what I call a "***cancer conditioning process***" that one apparently goes through. It works with a telescoping effect that enhances each stage on the cancer odyssey.

The first stage of the cancer conditioning process is true panic.

It's when one realizes that one is confronted with cancer. That's only natural and, believe it or not, a *healthy* reaction since almost everyone is programmed to believe that cancer is a 'death sentence' and you are not ready for it. That's not the case. The *real* issue is the body is saying that its biochemistry is screwed up with toxins and needs to be detoxified and revitalized. What cancer patients in reality don't hear are the real-life stories of those who fought cancer and won using non-toxic treatments. Only conventional treatments are lauded after the five-year-survival-rate-cancer-free watershed mark is reached, often only to experience a secondary cancer. Please consider the following information from a government website detailing *NEW MALIGNANCIES FOLLOWING BREAST CANCER*.

> *In the current SEER study, women treated with radiotherapy had marginally higher risks of developing a subsequent breast tumor than nonirradiated women.*

Cyclophophamide-anthracycline-based regimens, in wider use in recent years, may be associated with higher leukemia risks, but in absolute terms the risk appears low when standard doses are administered (cumulative incidence less than 0.5% at 8-10 years) (Smith et al, 2003).

Radiation also appeared to contribute to the elevated risk of cancers of the esophagus, bone, and soft tissue among long-term survivors of breast cancer, with higher risks observed among irradiated patients compared with nonirradiated patients. The heightened risk of esophageal cancer was evident 5 years or more after radiation treatment, and risk rose to nearly 3-fold among 10-year survivors (O/E=2.93, O=28). [44]

So doesn't it make sense to use non-toxic methods of repairing and fortifying the immune system, which are the most effective modalities for dealing with any cancer in the body? That is key in holistic cancer treatment, not a further compromise of the immune system and liver from toxic chemotherapy— why do you lose your hair—and why do liver enzymes have to be monitored? Not only because of possible liver metastasis, but also because toxicity levels need to be monitored—similar monitoring goes on when the prescription drug Coumadin [Warfarin—rat poison] is prescribed as a blood thinner.

The second stage of the cancer conditioning process is sorting out what you, the patient, want and how you want to be treated.

And not necessarily what your family, friends, or doctors want, or push on you. It will be you—and only you—who will have to endure and suffer the treatments, which often are horrendous, disfiguring, and never-ending.

The third stage of the cancer conditioning process is acceptance.

Okay, so I have it—now I have to beat it. In my opinion, the worst thing a patient can do is dwell on the stage of cancer she has. That creates negative vibrations—along with fear and worries—that affect health and healing. Acceptance doesn't mean that you roll over and do nothing. It means that you realistically understand what's going on in your body and make the necessary changes to lifestyle and obtain treatment *you want for your body.*

For some, that protocol may be surgery-radiation-chemotherapy. That's *your* decision. However, without proper dietary changes and nutritional support, plus detoxification of the liver and body, your immune system most likely will fail you and that leads to more toxic doses of radiation and chemo, often with resultant secondary cancers.

The fourth stage of the cancer conditioning process is commitment.

The commitment a cancer patient has to make is more than a hundred percent because your body is now depending upon you to do right by it to get well. Your body will respond—to give an astrological analogy—*when all the stars are in proper alignment,* so to speak. That means that you've set your course and are determined to make it work to get the most benefits out of each modality in your protocol, no matter what it takes.

And, there probably is a fourth sub-stage to the cancer conditioning process evolving, I think. That's when conventional breast cancer treatments aren't working for you; you are getting worse or given a few weeks to live; or you just can't tolerate the adverse effects of conventional cancer treatments any longer. That's when most people seek out alternative or holistic treatments. That, too, is when they push the restart button at stage two above. However, that's also when a tidal shift occurs not only in thinking but also with recalibration of treatment using holistic therapies. I've heard about and seen that happen so many times that I've come to believe the fourth sub-stage of the cancer conditioning process is becoming the norm for many cancer patients recently.

To help breast cancer patients with understanding and working through the 'Psycho-Bio-Physiological Chemistry' that surrounds cancer, I heartily suggest your checking out Chapter 35, *Information Resources*.

A better understanding of the body-mind connection in breast cancer and its treatment comes out of the protocols of Dr Sylvia Flesner, ND, whose work has been discussed in detail in the book, *Recaging the Beast, The Disease Behind Disease: The Yeast-Fungal Connection,* for which I had the privilege of being the author's editor and writing consultant during the manuscript phase of that book.

In Chapter 14, *The Body-Mind Connection*, Jane Remington, the author, details one of the more—if not the most—important aspects that deals with releasing the psychological features and effects of cancer, that is the letting go of whatever is *eating you up inside*, e.g., past grievances, hurts, unresolved life issues, plus coming to the ultimate resolve—forgiveness and release. There's a powerful mental exercise and homework assignment that both Jane and Dr Flesner prescribe that, after having completed it with all honesty, allows one to get on with the healing process. I heartily recommend *Recaging the Beast*; it's an awesome book available on Amazon.com.

Perhaps the body-mind connection and forgiveness with release are nothing new. In one of the early books (*Sirach* 28, second century BCE) of the Bible there is reference to what Jane and Dr Flesner point out, and that is:

Could anyone nourish anger against another and expect healing from the Lord?

To which I'd like to add that humans also ought to establish an *attitude of gratitude*. Be grateful for *everything* because everything in life is for a reason, even though we may not realize it at the time. Expressing gratitude, I think, is another form of release—a release that blesses all involved.

Furthermore, to get well one has to be willing to *divest oneself of baggage* that one has been carrying around for a while—sometimes years or even lifetimes. When we can forgive and forget, our cells will be able to do the very same thing. Cells—natural killer (NK) cells, in particular—do have a capacity for memory. That sounds so esoteric, I know, but science is recognizing that fact, and there should be no reason to hold a grudge even at cellular levels, I truly believe. Talk to your cells; tell them how much you love them and want them to be healthy and well. It just may work.

Do some fun thing for the kid in you everyday.

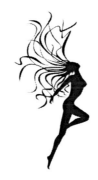

Chapter Six
The Immune System
A Different *Observation of Its Role in Disease and Healing*

Understanding the laws of nature does not mean that we are immune to their operations.

... David Gerrold
American writer (1944—)

*T*rying to discuss the human immune system is like trying to cover an elephant with a handkerchief—there's just too much territory and too little capability, particularly in this book where space is limited and the reader may not want to know all there is to know.

Having presented that caveat, here's what I think you may want—or need—to know about the immune system in your quest for overcoming breast cancer. At minimum, I hope it will help you understand the whys and wherefores of what is done in the name of holistic healing.

The immune system is made up of various cells: B-cells, T-cells, and Natural Killer (NK) cells called lymphocytes (they identify 'enemy cells' and attack) and macrophages (surround a foreign organism 'enemy' and kill it usually by 'eating' it). Both lymphocytes and macrophages are produced within human bone marrow. Foreign enemies include harmful organisms or tissue growths. T-lymphocytes kill infected cells; B-lymphocytes produce antibodies against infection. Furthermore, plasma cells, located in bone marrow, are the principal source of antibodies, one of the primary controls of foreign microorganisms.

First and foremost, the immune system also includes numerous bodily organs and systems that fall back upon each other, so to speak. [45] *The immune system is holistic!*

Most of our immune system 'resides' in the human intestinal tract where microorganisms do a Herculean job keeping us healthy when we have a healthful flora composition. Those microorganisms are known as *microflora* and can get out of hand rather easily, especially from antibiotic and birth control pill use, heavy-duty drugs like prednisone, alcoholic beverages, sweets and sodas, vinegar and vinegar-based condiments and salad dressings, and yeasted breads and pastries. I can hear your exasperation now: *"What is she talking about?"*

All those things tend to kill off the friendly or good microflora we need in our gut while they 'fertilize' the harmful or 'bad' ones like *Candida Albicans*, which compromise our immune system—and us—if you can believe that. I'd like to share some bodily symptoms, signs, or clues that *candida* may be compromising your immune system.

- Vaginal/yeast infections
- Need to use panty liners because of wetness—that's *candida* in the vagina walls sweating, especially after eating foods that 'excite' them.
- In men, it's jock itch
- Nail fungus—either fingernails, or most commonly, toenails
- Food cravings, especially starches, sweets, candy, chocolate, sodas, and sugary foods that feed yeast and candida, as they are hungry critters that love to eat and multiply.

Candida Albicans is the most common fungus among us. Even though we need a proper balance of it within our gut for digestion and elimination, *overgrowth* becomes a health problem that impacts the immune system more than allopathic medicine tends to realize at this point in time of medical science, I truly feel. Unfortunately, chemotherapy promotes the rapid growth of *candida.* Eva Roberts discusses chemo, yeast and fungus in her article "Does Chemo Kill Yeast & Fungus?" [46] It's a worthwhile read to understand how what you put into your mouth impacts your immune system.

There are two simultaneous ways to attack *candida* to bring it under control and into balance:

- A 100 percent *yeast-free* diet. Please consider reading the book *Recaging the Beast* available on Amazon.com, and
- Daily use of megaflora probiotic supplements that contain several strains of *lactobacillus, bifidobacterium,* and *streptococcus.*

In my opinion there is no better resource on that than Jane Remington's book, *Recaging the Beast*, for which I was Jane's writing consultant and manuscript editor.

At this time rather than rehashing the need for transforming your diet from yeast promoting to *yeast-free,* may I refer you, please, to various chapters in Part II of this book on food, diet, and nutrition. Those chapters [14-34] will inform you how to switch from a basic yeast-fungus-promoting eating pattern most people eat today to a *totally delicious yeast-free* diet.

For those who want *to really go after the 'beast'*, there's more that you can do:

- Drink *Pao D'Arco* tea, at least two 8 oz. cups daily.
- Supplement your regimen with a teaspoon or two of dried wheat grass in water or *freshly pressed green* vegetable juice to help alkalize the body's pH thereby assisting in killing off *candida.* I found using a stick blender helps to emulsify dried wheat grass in liquids. Keep dried wheat grass powder in your freezer.
- A *substitute* for dried wheat grass is *liquid organic chlorophyll* from organic alfalfa. Keep it in your refrigerator.

- Eliminate all mushrooms from the diet, as they are the fruiting bodies of fungi.
- Cheeses, particularly hard cheese, tend to produce molds—that green or black stuff you find on cheese you forgot about in the refrigerator. I suggest not eating cheese until you are well again because of its mold-producing capability and spores in hard cheeses, in particular.

When you realize that your food cravings have stopped, your panties aren't wet anymore, and you may be losing unwanted weight, you will begin to understand just how important "recaging the beast" really is.

It is my opinion, and that of others who have gone this route, once you get *candida* under control, you should stay on a *daily maintenance* megaflora probiotic dose for the rest of your life. As I see it, it can't hurt and only helps to keep the immune system healthy and capable of shooting down any cancer cells that may come our way almost daily from our modern, chemicalized lifestyles. There seems to be no way of getting away from toxic chemicals anymore.

However, there is one more thing you can do to jump-start the immune system, I think, and that's going on a detox program that will eliminate toxins from body tissue and cells.

In my case I couldn't get on a detox fast enough because of having been exposed to toxic fumes twice, formaldehyde, and neighbors' herbicides even though I did all I could over the years trying to eliminate toxins from my body.

Toxic chemicals, in particular, have an affinity for storing in fatty tissue, even though you may not be overweight. Humans have what I call 'fat bumpers'—or what in medical terminology is called 'essential body fat'—around internal organs, which protect them from bruising. Nevertheless, within that 'good' fat is where chemical toxins store and must be detoxified, if we are to overcome cancer. I cannot impress upon you how important it is to rid the body of toxic chemicals because they do prevent body chemistry from functioning optimally. So knowing that, I chose a liquid homeopathic detox program whose drops I drank in a pint of water over the course of the day for about six weeks. I did four rounds of *Guna Biotherapeutics Detox Treatment* (<gunainc.com>) while writing this book. Personally, I can tell you that *Guna* really got stuff that had been deep within my body. Even my managing physician was impressed with the results.

I cannot tell you how much I began to sweat—my body was eliminating toxins without a sauna—plus the body odor that manifested. Whew! I went from no B.O.—don't use antiperspirants or deodorants—to wow! Where'd that come from? Detox was working and my body—neck, torso, underarms, and thighs—was sweating while cleansing hard-to-release toxins that apparently were deep within my body's tissues.

Also, I increased my intake of vitamin D to optimize my blood levels of that important immune-building vitamin. There are in-home vitamin D test kits that I discourage your using. Talk to your holistic physician about running a vitamin D blood test that will give you several readings on various levels of vitamin D, since research is showing that low levels of *serum* vitamin D have been linked with breast cancer. Vitamin D "arms" the immune system to do battle fighting disease(s).

Take the time to remind yourself that you are not the general manager of the universe.

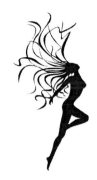

Chapter Seven
Whom or What Can We Trust?

No science is immune to the infection of
politics and the corruption of power.

… Jacob Bronowski, PhD (1908—1974)
A Polymath / Author, *The Ascent of Man*

The intent of this book—and this chapter, in particular—is not to castigate but to point out an analogy to what Shylock said in Shakespeare's *Hamlet*, Act 1, Scene 3:

There are more things in heaven and earth, Horatio,
than are dreamt of in your philosophy.

Modern medicine, pharmacology—and chemotherapy for cancer, in particular—believe *they* should be the only modalities that legally can provide information, services, and products. Notwithstanding, allopathic medicine can be equated with Shakespeare's Horatio, I think.

Conventional medicine does not want to stretch itself to embrace the holistic healing arts, many of which have come down through generations—if not eons of time, in some instances, e.g., acupuncture and herbology. Modern medicine considers itself the pinnacle of the healing arts, yet fails numerous people in so many ways, if not by chance, probably by flawed science and technology that are used almost as bludgeons against time-tested and honored healing traditions of natural healthcare. Again, I must ask the question, "How did humans make it for so long without modern medicine?"

If you think about that remark, you ought to wonder why two trades—basically medical doctors and their union, the American Medical Association, and the pharmaceutical industry—were capable of establishing a monopoly that seems to be falling flat on its face despite its propaganda, media spin, and congressional, federal, and state health agency manipulations to maintain draconian healthcare control via mandates and legislation. One prime example is vaccinations; another is health insurance reimbursement for only allopathic cancer treatments and medications, not holistic practices, which are much less expensive and equally effective. When allopaths give up on cancer patients, where do those patients go? Holistic cancer care.

The above is not an indictment, but reality. Healthcare consumers may not know because of unawareness, manipulation of information via the media, which is controlled, or fear—something medicine relies upon to keep you in their camp, just listen to radio and TV advertisements. Technological advances often can border on torment, e.g., repeated rounds of chem-otherapy and/or radiotherapy including the new *CyberKnife* as their 'gold standard treatments'. What amuses me, quite frankly, are seemingly self-righteous 'puffery' advertisements whereby they try to sound like they really care while you can envision cash registers going caching, caching, caching! Their cancer treatments aren't cheap, even though health insurance pays for most of them. I've heard stories of cancer patients who have had so many 'gold standard treatments' that insurance companies are declining paying for additional treatments.

Technology, of which the medical arts certainly is an aspect, includes the pharmaceutical industry and other ancillary industries dealing with health and healthcare issues. Because conventional doctors apparently have bought into Big Pharma's "Emperor's New Clothes" spin-tale propaganda and hype, I think MDs truly are more scared than consumers know because MDs don't want to lose their *sacred peer status*, so they must keep perpetuating holistic cancer treatment putdowns plus lauding practices that lead to higher and higher healthcare costs, more and more iatrogenic illnesses, severe adverse reactions from prescription medications that aren't cheap, plus a plethora of chronic diseases once the bane of old age, now the daily plight of young children.

To illustrate the above, I'd like to share some concerns that may not be apparent to healthcare consumers, which can color one's thinking when known.

1. *"The vast majority of drugs—more than 90 percent—only work in 30 to 50 percent of the people."* Who said that?

It's been attributed to none other than Dr Allen Roses, then Vice President of Genetics at GlaxoSmithKline in 2003.

Dr Roses is quoted further with saying, *"Drugs for Alzheimer's disease work in fewer than one in three patients, whereas those for cancer are only effective in a quarter of patients. Drugs for migraines, for osteoporosis, and arthritis work in about half the patients."* Perhaps we should take Dr Roses' statement at face value since he's an academic geneticist from Duke University. Furthermore, with only a quarter of cancer drugs effective, is there some kind of crapshoot going on?

2. *In the United States your odds of being killed by conventional medicine are 20 times greater than being killed in an automobile accident and almost 30 times greater than being killed by a gun!*

3. Listen to the frustration that some MDs experience because of having to follow the establishment's edicts. *"I want to do more for my patients than what's offered by the pharmaceutical industry because I realized earlier on that modern medicine has become, unfortunately, more of a big business than a healing science."* Paul Beals, MD, CCN, Georgetown University School of Medicine (Course Instructor 1996-2004: *Introduction to Complementary and Alternative Medicine*)

4. According to the *Archives of Internal Medicine*, Vol. 171, No. 16, September 12, 2011 article "Less Is More: Communicating Uncertainties About Prescription

Drugs to the Public," *Conclusions* section stated, *A substantial proportion of the public mistakenly believes that the FDA approves only extremely effective drugs and drugs lacking serious side effects.* **However, there also is a caveat offered by one of the study's authors, and it is this: FDA approval means that only** *"the benefits are judged to be greater than the harms."* **Do you want to read that again? Apparently nothing is mentioned about safety and efficacy.**

5. According to a September 2010 Centers for Disease Control and Prevention (CDC) report, nearly 90 percent of adults in the month before the report, reported taking prescription drugs. Close to 75 percent of senior citizens take two or more prescription drugs, while 37 percent take *five or more*!

   It's been noted that senior citizens who take multiple prescription drugs are at high risks for falls. As high as 15 percent of drug interactions or adverse events can result in deaths.

   Do we have a 'legal' drug culture prescribed by MDs to profit Big Pharma, who in turn pays kickbacks or commissions to MDs for writing 'mucho' scripts for prescriptions? If you don't believe that happens, please read a fabulous book, *The Risks of Prescription Drugs,* Donald W Light, PhD, Ed., Columbia University Press, available on Amazon.com.

6. The FDA posted a safety alert September 2, 2011, warning about the risk of kidney failure for the drug *Reclast*

(zoledronic acid), an osteoporosis drug. To understand drug safety issues, you may want to read the FDA's information posted about Reclast's recall. [47]

If you or anyone you love or know has suffered adverse events from medication, the Food and Drug Administration (FDA) has an online website, *MedWatch*, where you can report adverse reactions. You can access it at <accessdata. fda.gov/scripts/medwatch/medwatch-online.htm>. Some think this CDC reporting system may act like the pharmaceutical industry's safety and efficacy studies done *post marketing.*

7. Last but not least, may I introduce the nasty side of what I call the 'politics of health' that, in my opinion, keep allopathy and its muse, Big Pharma, predatory? *Dirty tricks and smear campaigns.* Please read Chapter 8, *The Fitzgerald Report,* documenting antics against holistic cancer treatments in the 1950s. A more recent episode involved the 'sacred cow' of pharmacology and medicine—vaccines—wherein Dr Andrew Wakefield, a well-respected British medical doctor, had an article published June 1998 in the *British Medical Journal* (BMJ), and upon a journalist's apparently fabricated story he pursued, got a BMJ retraction of Wakefield's article in January 2011 that has professionally eviscerated the doctor. To understand what happened, you may want to read about it at *Natural News* <natural-news.com/033516_BMJ_financial_ties.html>. [48] The

aforementioned website tells about *BMJ's secret finan-cial ties* to vaccine maker Merck pharmaceuticals during the publication of articles attacking Dr Wakefield.

Oh what games they play!

So, whom or what can we trust? There's some pretty serious stuff that goes on while healthcare consumers willingly place their lives and bodies into conventional healthcare hands, not knowing what could happen, and for which many have paid the price with ruined lives.

According to the website *Your Medical Detective,* [49] there are:

106,000 *deaths per year* from negative effects of drugs

80,000 *deaths per year* from infections in hospitals

45,000 *deaths per year* from other errors in hospitals

12,000 *deaths per year* from unnecessary surgery

7,000 *deaths per year* from medication errors in hospitals

A whopping 250,000 deaths per year and no one is held accountable or goes to jail.

Unfortunately, cancer management is one area where that can happen more often and is the reason that everyone who contracts that disease is scared skinny. It's because of conven-tional medicine's poor track record and patients' horror sto-ries about undergoing cancer treatments that bridles patients' minds and scares the living crap out of us. Conventional medi-cine, in my opinion, has a license to do that legally, and is not held accountable or liable for lost lives to failing cancer treatments, and still gets reimbursed *handsomely* by health insurance plans. Is there any wondering why I opted for holistic cancer management?

Over the years of being a healthcare professional and researcher into patient issues, I've heard at least a hundred or more pathetically sad stories of how oncologists told patients,

"There's nothing more we can do; get your affairs in order." Left bereft with totally toxic bodies from radiation and numerous rounds of chemotherapy, patients and their families hit the panic button and, in their desperation, turn to holistic cancer treatments where they find compassionate care and are not turned away. Many patients too often are so toxic that they do succumb under holistic care where, unfortunately, a stigma of harm is attributed rather than to the actual 'killing fields' of radiation and chemotherapy.

However, I cannot tell you how many stories I've heard of cancer patients—even stage four patients—regaining health again from holistic cancer therapies. I also cannot tell you how many human interest stories that have been told to me about people on prescription medications who got fed up and went off them on their own only to find lower blood pressure readings, decreases in blood sugar levels that kept them in the 'diabetes' range with medication for it, and even patients in hospice care who recovered after deciding they wanted no more medication if they were going to die anyway.

So again, I must ask, *"Whom or what can we trust?"*

Before I leave the topic of *whom or what can we trust*, I'd like to share that anyone who had a polio vaccine as a child in the 1950s through the 1970s may be at special risk for any type of cancer, including breast cancer, due to the presence of SV40 and cancer in the polio vaccine. You don't believe that? Well, if you turn to *Appendix A* in the back of this book and read my article "The 'Unknown' About Polio Vaccine: SV40 and Cancer" published April 9, 2011 on the Internet at *VacTruth. com*, you will be very surprised at what you read, including that the U.S. Congress held a hearing September 10, 2003, wherein the conclusion was:

> *There is no dispute that millions of Americans received polio vaccines that were contaminated with the virus called Simian Virus 40, or SV–40. There also is no dispute that SV–40 is capable of causing cancer, but there is a major dispute as to how many Americans may have received the contaminated vaccine, with estimates ranging from 4 million to 100 million people. There is also a major dispute as to when the polio vaccine supply got cleaned up. In addition, nobody knows how many people got sick or died because of the contaminated vaccines.*

Furthermore, the 'patriarch of vaccines' at Merck, Dr Maurice Hilleman, MD, candidly spoke on camera about what is in vaccines that you may want to check out for yourself by viewing <youtube.com/watch?v=4W2MJbcgn1g>. [50]

In view of that alarming factual information, most adults today need to be vigilant and 'proactive' about keeping themselves as free from free radical production in the body as possible, since DNA damage can become 'cumulative' and bingo—cancer!

Chapter 34, *Holistic PREVENTIVE Measures To Avoid Breast Cancer,* offers helpful suggestions for everyone at any age as to what they can do to reduce the risks of developing any form of cancer and, in particular, breast cancer for both women and men.

Before I leave this topic of *whom or what can we trust,* there's something that I think you ought to know that maybe—just maybe—will encourage you to think for yourself about what's being presented to you in the name of science. This has to deal with food—chickens in particular—that ought to make you wonder about the food-cancer connection.

Poultry farmers—other than organic growers—have counted on a pharmaceutical, *Roxarsone®,* to treat parasites in chickens they raise in high-rise hen house 'condominiums' where animal droppings fall down on chickens below, plus all sorts of unhealthy living conditions for any animal, especially chickens who Nature designed to obtain immune building organisms from pecking in the soil and grass.

Researchers proved that Roxarsone prompts *angiogenesis* in human cells, which is the process that tumor cells use to supply blood so that tumors can grow. Are you ready for this? Two million pounds of Roxarsone used to be added to chicken feed *each year! Roxarsone is a source of arsenic—a toxin, poison, and probable carcinogen when it interacts with other chemicals in the body.* How much non-organically-grown chicken have you eaten?

The European Union *banned* Roxarsone in 1999, while the U.S. USDA/FDA kept approving it for chicken husbandry in the USA. Only in June 2011 did the FDA announce that Roxarsone would no longer be sold in the USA. Again, we have to ask, "*Whom or what can you trust?*" Apparently the FDA may have been more concerned with the profits Alpharma, a Pfizer subsidiary, would make rather than the health of U.S. consumers and the safety of the food supply. Or, were Alpharma's lobbyists so convincing, plus Big Pharma's contributions that subsidize FDA operations due to Congress's cut backs in funding, much more important than the health and welfare of citizens those agencies are supposed to be in business to protect? This is the very tip of the proverbial iceberg on chemicals in the food supply. It ought to convince you of the importance of eating organically grown food.

Another aspect regarding food safety is what the U.S. Food and Drug Administration claims about seafood from the Gulf of Mexico after the oil spill of April 11, 2010, and the millions of gallons of Corexit pumped into the Gulf to disperse the oil.

According to the article "Seafood Contamination After the BP Gulf Oil Spill and Risks to Vulnerable Populations: A Critique of the FDA Risk Assessment" in the journal *Environmental Health Perspective*, authors Ellman and Solomon studied available Poly Aromatic Hydrocarbons (PAHs) testing data for shellfish after the spill. Ellman says up to 53 percent of the shrimp tested had PAH levels *"exceeding our revised levels of concern for pregnant women who eat a lot of Gulf shellfish."* They also question the vulnerability for a developing fetus. [51]

So how can we trust federal agencies to protect us from contaminated fish and seafood that contain PAHs, known carcinogens?

To add to the proverbial *insult to injury theme*, consider this advertising out of yesteryear. The Soda Pop Board of America crafted an advertisement touting this:

> *For a better start in life, start cola earlier! How soon is too soon? Not soon enough. Laboratory tests over the last few years have proven that babies who start drinking soda during that early formative period have a much higher chance of gaining acceptance and "fitting in" during those awkward pre-teen and teen years. So, do yourself a favor. Start them on a strict regimen of sodas and other sugary carbonated beverages right now, for a lifetime of guaranteed happiness.*

Do you believe that? I have the ad in my computer files along with the graphics that accompanied the text. How insane, in my opinion, since dependency upon sugary foods is a known factor leading to childhood and adult diabetes. How bizarre in light of today's warnings about sugary soft drinks.

Endocrinologists who conducted studies on teens and sodas found that

A single 12-oz sugar-sweetened beverage per day translates to about 1 pound of weight gain over 3 to 4 weeks. [52]

Science knows that weight gain plays a role in the etiology of cancer. But look at what the Soda Pop Board ads were saying years ago. So again, whom or what can we trust?

Remember my discussion earlier in the book about pH and its relationship to cancer. Well, many sodas have a pH value of 2.5, which is very acidic and the same pH value as vinegar. Would you drink a can of vinegar? Furthermore, soda's high levels of phosphorus leach calcium both from the bones thereby setting up soda drinkers for a proclivity to broken bones, and from teeth enamel by erosion causing dental problems. Diet soda is worse nutritionally because of the synthetic sugars that play havoc with the endocrine system and tend to add on pounds faster than real sugar.

Even Cancer Support Groups Need Questioning

Applause and kudos to *Breast Cancer Action,* a national advocacy group located in San Francisco, California, for their courage to expose a dichotomy of sorts in groups that sell products to raise funds for research. Here's an example:

> *Pinkwashing has reached a new low this year with Promise Me, a perfume commissioned by Susan G. Komen for the Cure. Promise Me contains chemicals not listed in the ingredients that: a) are regulated as toxic and hazardous, b) have not been adequately evaluated for human safety, and c) have demonstrated negative health effects.* [53]

At Breast Cancer Action, we call that pinkwashing, and we urge you to Raise a Stink! With us about it. If you visit their website <thinkbeforeyoupink.org/> you will find an action link about raising a stink.

Also from *Breast Cancer Action's* website:

• *70 percent of people with breast cancer have none of the known risk factors.*

• *Non-industrialized countries have lower breast cancer rates than industrialized countries. People who move to industrialized countries from countries with low rates develop the same breast cancer rates of the industrialized country.*

• *Estrogen is a hormone closely linked with the development of breast cancer. Numerous synthetic chemicals act like estrogen in our bodies, including common weed killers and pesticides, plastic additives or by-products, ingredients in spray paints and paint removers, and polyvinyl chloride (PVC) used extensively in the manufacture of food packaging as well as in medical products, appliances, cars, toys, credit cards and rainwear.*

• *Ionizing radiation from x-rays and nuclear waste is a proven cause of breast cancer.*

• *A growing body of evidence from exprimental, body burden and ecological research indicates that there is a connection between envrionmental factors and breast cancer. There are over 85,000 synthetic chemicals on the marrket today, from preservatives in our lipstick to flame retardants in our sofas, from plasticizers in our water bottles to pesticides on our fruits and vegetables. The U.S. government has no adequate chemical regulation policy, therefore companies are allowed to manufacture and use chemicals without ever establishing their safety. As the use of chemicals has risen in the U.S. and other industralized countries, so have rates of breast and other cancers.* [53]

Breast Cancer Action seems to have the facts about breast cancer correct and which I discuss in depth in my last book, *Our Chemical Lives And The Hijacking Of Our DNA, A Probe Into What's Probably Making Us Sick*, available on Amazon. com. Also, *BCA* is vocal about the role of chemicals in cancer, which I applaud wholeheartedly. I don't think any cancer advocacy group should compromise health and values, even to raise money for research—but that's my opinion.

One More Example to Prove the Point

The Center for Science in the Public Interest filed a class action lawsuit October 14, 2011, against food processor General Mills for deceptive and false advertising regarding 'healthy claims' for *Fruit Roll-Ups, Fruit by the Foot,* and *Fruit Gushers* because ads claim those products are healthier than they really are. See ingredient contents as per CSPI's legal brief filed:

> *"In fact, Defendant's Fruit Snacks contained trans fat, added sugars, and artificial food dyes; lacked significant amounts of real, natural fruit; and had no dietary*

fiber. Thus, although the Products were marketed as being healthful and nutritious for children and adults alike, selling these Fruit Snacks was little better than giving candy to children," per the complaint filed with the court.

For readers who want to know more about that class action lawsuit, here's where to access the pdf file with the complaint <cspinet.org/new/pdf/fruit_roll-ups_complaint .pdf>.

With all the examples of apparently confusing or often 'retracted' (mis)information regarding health I've presesnted, it's not difficult to understand that there is a ton of misleading information out there regarding not only breast cancer treatment but the very food we need for bodies to be healthy and/ or get well. That information needs to be weighed intelligently by a woman who finds herself confronted with breast cancer. Those often 'Pinocchio-type' messages are called 'corporate spin'—some claim 'corporate sin'—to sell products or services. The medical profession by no means is exempt either, in my opinion, especially pharmaceutical makers who sell chemotherapy at thousands of dollars per treatment, even if health insurance pays for it. Whom or what can you trust? You, the patient, have to decide for yourself, as it will be you—and only you—who will have to live with the consequences.

Health truly is wealth!

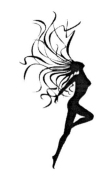

Chapter Eight
The Fitzgerald Report

The Official Report to the U.S. Senate Interstate
Commerce Committee
August 3, 1953
[Alternative Cancer Treatment Harassment]

We must not tolerate oppressive government or industrial oligarchy
in the form of monopolies and cartels.

... Henry A Wallace (1888—1965)
33rd Vice President of the USA

To understand the politics of cancer and why there is no official cure found for cancer after all these years, *I think* it is important to review some of the histrionics surrounding cancer treatment as documented in the official *Fitzgerald Report*. Nevertheless, in all the years since that *Report*, X-rays (mammograms), surgery, radiation, and chemotherapy have remained the 'gold standard' with very little, if any, innovative *non-toxic allopathic* treatments sanctioned and reimbursed by health insurance policies. As of 2007 a *Billion Dollars* had been spent on BREAST cancer research alone. What does that tell you?

> *Since 1946 it is said that the American Cancer Society has invested over $2 billion in research trying to find a cure. Several sources claim that between $10-12 million a year is spent by the ACS in the state of California alone. The NCI is another institute said to spend around $5-6 million a year researching and trying to develop treatment for those effected* [sic] *by this disease.* [54]

The questions then, that this author is inspired to ask, are these: If they are spending that much money and getting nowhere, do they know what they are doing? Are they looking in the appropriate and correct areas of research? And, why would they want to dissuade medical doctors who come up with holistic/alternative cures and prosecute them? That doesn't seem to make sense if you really are looking for a cure. Now does it? Or is it a control issue, e.g., money?

Here is the link to the Fitzgerald Report.
<docs.google.con/viewer?a=v&q=cache:EnpGA7cxLy 4J:legacy.library.ucf.edu/dodumentStore/h/y/s/hys5aa00/ Shys5aa00.pdf+A+REPORT+TO+THE+SENATE+IN

TERTSTATE+COMMERCE+COMMITTEE+ON+T
HE+NEED+FOR+INVESTIGATION+OF+CANCER
&hl=en&gl=us&pid=bl&srcid=ADGEESgFoDG7Nsuq-
aWO6gRHbw-FL3pAqKw8k3QxC61T5HNenLi3Wy_
xbnNEftq6bZf4DeSDYQfuhkIsi9ZBMpXTvm9oOwX
hMN_-UOGuqjex0iblhFiUz23sWiBumLCOR34-rwgq1_
r0&sig=AHIEtbQTGW7Bo6NAEmtpxr-1R3BaFLzF6g>

Since the *Fitzgerald Report* is a document of public record and accessed at the above URL address, the author of this book decided to annotate it in italics so that readers can appreciate what's been going on seemingly for ages to destroy holistic non-toxic research, treatments, and cures for cancer.

Catherine J Frompovich's Annotation (*in italics*) to Excerpts From the *Fitzgerald Report*
Please note that I did not delete the typos and errors.

if radium, X-ray, or surgery or either of them is the complete answer, then the greatest hoax of the age is being perpetrated upon the people by the continued appeal for funds for further research. *CJF: Note that this was back in 1953 that appeals for donations to cancer research was questioned because Special Counsel Fitzgerald assessed that cancer treatments of X-ray, surgery, and radiation therapy were the answer in cancer treatments, which still is the 'gold standard' today, almost 60 years later.*

Because of fear or favor, are forced to line up with the so-called ac-ted view of the'Iinerican [American]

Medical Assol_qation, *[Association]* or should this commlttee make a full-scale investiga-tion of the organized ef ;Loxt o *[can't decipher]* hinder, suppress, and restrict the free flow of drugs which allegedly'have proven successful in cases where clinical records, case history, pathological reports, and :X-ray photographic proof, together with the alleged cured patients, are available .

CJF: Note that medical records and proof were availa-ble in 1953 documenting there were alternative non-toxic cures to cancer and they were being suppressed. Nothing has changed in almost 60 years.

Accordingly, we should determine whether exist-ing agencies, both public and private, are engaged in and have pursued a policy of harassment, ridicule, slan-der, and libelous attacks on others sincerely engaged in stamping out this curse of mankind.

CJF: Such activity has been accepted practice over the years with harassment of numerous medical doctors who have formulated alternative cancer cures. Some harassed physicians include Dr Emanuel Revici, MD, Dr Stanislaw R Burzynski, MD, PhD, William Donald Kelley, DDS, Dr Lawrence Burton, PhD, Dr Hans Nieper, MD, just to name a few.

My *[Special Counsel Fitzgerald's]* investigation to date should convince this committee that a conspir-acy does exist to stop the free flow and use of drugs in interstate commerce which allegedly have solid therapeutic value . Public and private funds have been thrown around like conf etti at a country fair to close up and destroy clinics, hospitals, and scientific research laboratories which do not conform to the vewpoint of medical associations .

CJF: This paragraph does not exaggerate what happened and continues to happen to this very day because of the influence of medical associations, lobbyists, and federal agency 'hit squads' out to destroy any type of holistic therapies, not just cancer treatments. In my opinion, such activity should be prosecuted legally under the Sherman Antitrust Act, which according to Wikipedia was the first Federal statute to limit cartels and monopolies, and today still forms the basis for most antitrust litigation by the United States federal government. After all, there seems to be one huge revolving door policy and monopoly that exists within medicine and the pharmaceutical industry, and it operates like a merry-go-round at the U.S. Food and Drug Administration, in my opinion.

Please take note of what *Special Counsel Fitzgerald said:* "My investigation to date should convince this committee that **a conspiracy does exist** to stop the free flow and use of drugs in interstate commerce which allegedly have solid therapeutic value." [CJF emphasis added]

The Fitzgerald Report, August 3, 1953
[as copied from the website] [55]

From : Benedict F. Fitzgerald, Jr., special counsel to the Committee on Interstate and Foreign Commerce.

To : Hon. JOHN W. BRICKER and members of the Interstate and Foreign Commerce Committee of the United States Senate.

Subject : Progress report on study requested by the late Senator Charles W. Tobey, chairman, Senate Interstate and Foreign Commerce Committee.

PROJECT

http://legacy.library.ucsf.edu/tid/hys5aa00/pdf

The undersigned, as special counsel to the Senate Interstate and Foreign Commerce Committee, was directed to supervise a study of the following :

1. All those individuals, organizations, foundations, hospitals and clinics, throughout the United States, which have an effect upon interstate commerce and which have been conducting researches, investigations, experiments and demonstrations relating to the cause, prevention, and methods of diagnosis and treatment of the disease cancer, to determine the interstate ramifications of their operations, their financial structures, including their fundraising methods, and the amounts expended for clinical research as distinguished from administrative expenditures, and to ascertain the extent

---

of the therapeutic value claimed by each in the use of its particular therapy.

2. The facts involving the discovery of, the imports from a foreign country of, the researches upon, and the interstate experiments, demonstrations, and use of the various drugs, preparations, and remedies for the treatment of the disease cancer, such drugs to include the so-called wonder drug krebiozen, gloxylide, mucorhicin, and others.

3. The facts involving the interstate conspiracy, if any, engaged in by any individuals, organizations, corporations, associatioris, and combines of any kind whatsoever, to hinder, suppress, or restrict the free flow or transmission of krebiozen, gloxylide, and mucorhicin, and other drugs, preparations and remedies, and information, researches, investigations, experiments and demonstrations relating to the cause, prevention and methods of diagnosis and treatment of the disease cancer.

. . .Thereafter, the undersigned traveled to Illinois to investigate the so-called krebiozen controversy, and on July 2, 1953, wrote a report on his findings which is attached hereto and marked "Exhibit A." Included in this report was the evaluation:

"The controversy is involved and requires further research and development. There is reason to believe that the AMA has been hasty, capricious, arbitrary, and outright dishonest, and of course if the doctrine of 'respondeat superior' is to be observed, the alleged machinations of Dr. J. J. Moore (for the past 10 years the treasurer of the AMA) could involve the AMA and others in an interstate conspiracy of alarming proportions.

"The principal witnesses who tell of Dr. Moore's rascality are Alberto Barreira, Argentine cabinet member, and his secretary, Anna D. Schmidt."

Thereafter, the undersigned visited other areas, interrogating medical men, and on July 14, 1953, wrote a further report. Included in this was the evaluation :

"Being vitally interested and having tried to listen and observe closely, it is my profound conviction that this substance krebiozen is one of the most promising materials yet isolated for the management of cancer. It is biologically active. I have gone http://legacy.library.ucsf.edu/tid/hys5aa00/pdf over the records of 530 cases, most of them conducted at a distance from Chicago, by unbiased cancer experts and clinics. In reaching my conclusions I have of course discounted my own lay observations and relied mostly on the opinions of qualified canced research workers and ordinary experienced physicians.

"I have concluded that in the value of present cancer research, this substance and the theory behind it deserves the most full and complete and scientific study. Its value in the management of the cancer patient has been demonstrated in a sufficient number and per centage of cases to demand further work.

"Behind and over all this is the weirdest conglomeration of corrupt motives, intrigue, selfishness, jealousy, obstruction, and conspiracy that I have ever seen.

"Dr. Andrew C. Ivy, who has been conducting research upon this drug, is absolutely honest intellectually, scientifically, and in every other way. Moreover, he appears to be one of the most competent and unbiased cancer experts that I have ever come in contact with, having served on the board of the American Cancer Society and the American Medical Association, and in that capacity having been called upon to evaluate various types of cancer therapy. Dr. George 0. Stoddard, president of the University of Illinois, in assisting in the cessation of Dr. Ivy's research on cancer at the University of-Illinois, and in recommending the abolishment of the latter's post as vice president of that in5titution, has, in my opinion, shown attributes of intolerance for scientific research in general."

It is a matter of common knowledge that the entire subject matter is highly controversial and thus further and additional research and development would entail more time. A controversy among renowned surgeons, pathologists, cancerologists, and radiologists should not deter or silence this committee from carrying out the mandate contemplated and expressly directed by the late chairman of your committee, Senator Charles W. Tobey, by virtue of the resolution passed by the Senate.

. . .I have approached this problem with an open mind. Recognizing the importance of men skilled in the science of medicine, who are best informed, if not qualified, on the queston of cancer, its causes and treatment, I directed my attention to the propaganda by the American Medical Association and the American Cancer Society to the effect, namely, "that radium, X-ray therapy, and surgery are the only recognized treatments for cancer."

Is there any dispute among recognized medical scientists in America and elsewhere in the world on the use of radium and X-ray therapy in the treatment of cancer? The answer is definitely "Yes." There is a division of opinion on the use of radium and X-ray. Both agencies are destructive, not constructive. In the alleged destructtion of the abnormal, outlaw, or cancer cells both X-ray therapy and radium destroy normal tissue and normal cells. Recognized medical authorities in America and elsewhere state positively that X-ray therapy can cause cancer in and of itself. Documented cases are available.

http://legacy.library.ucsf.edu/tid/hys5aa00/pdf

The increased number of cancer patients in America of all ages and the apparent failure to presently cope with this dread disease indicates the necessity of a sustained effort of private and Federal agencies to continue research in the field of cancer, its causes and treatment. if radium, X-ray, or surgery or either of them is the complete answer, then the greatest hoax of the age is being perpetrated upon the people by the continued appeal for funds for further research.

If neither X-ray, radium, or surgery is the complete answer to this dreaded disease, and I submit that it is not, then what is the plain duty of society? Should we stand still? Should we sit idly by and count the number of physicians, surgeons, and cancerologists who are not. only divided but who, because of fear or favor, are forced to line up with the so-called ac-ted view of the'Iinerican Medical Assol_qation, or should this commlttee make a full-scale investigation of the organized ef ;Loxt to hinder, suppress, and restrict the free flow of drugs which allegedly'have proven successful in cases where clinical records, case history, pathological reports, and :X-ray photographic proof, together with the alleged cured patients, are available.

Accordingly, we should determine whether existing agencies, both public and private, are engaged in and have pursued a policy of harassment, ridicule, slander, and libelous attacks on others sincerely engaged in stamping out this curse of mankind. Have medical associations, through their officers, agents, servants and employees engaged in this practice? My investigation to date should convince this committee that a conspiracy does exist to stop the free flow and use of drugs in interstate commerce which allegedly have solid therapeutic value. Public and private funds have been thrown around like conf etti at a country fair to close up and destroy clinics, hospitals, and scientific research laboratories which do not conform to the vewpoint of medical associations.

. . . May I, with propriety, call your attention to the tragedy which has invaded the United States Senate. Four great Americans, all of them - Senator McMahon, Senator Wherry, Senator Vandenberg, and Senator Bob Taft - were all stricken down with this dreaded disease. We are under a compelling moral obligation to the memory of these great public servants and to the untold millions of cancer sufferers throughout the world to carry on this investigation. We cannot do otherwise.

Respectfully submitted.

Benedict F. Fitzgerald,

Special Counsel.

This Author's Comment:

If Special Counsel Fitzgerald candidly reported in 1953, *"Behind and over all this is the weirdest conglomeration of corrupt motives, intrigue, selfishness, jealousy, obstruction, and conspiracy that I have ever seen."*

then I, who have been researching consumer health issues for 35 years and counting, plus having been a registered lobbyist with the U.S. Congress for five years representing holistic healthcare issues, in addition to doing government relations and media work for holistic healthcare industry clients before federal agencies for several years, am left with nothing that leads me to believe things have changed, particularly in the cancer arena. However, I do believe that many healthcare issues have surfaced during subsequent years that would entice Special Counsel Benedict F Fitzgerald to investigate in 2012.

I know that remark is not very complimentary to the medical profession and its ancillary professions and businesses, but if I want to be as candid as Counsel Fitzgerald was in 1953, I must report what my experiences and research have taught and shown me.

What you don't know can affect you directly.

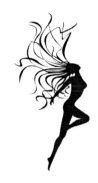

Chapter Nine
Radiation: What Is It?

My main frustration is the fear of cancer from low dose radiation, even by radiologists.

… **John R Cameron, PhD (1922—2005)**
Founder of nuclear medicine laboratory in UW Hospitals, 1959

To help understand what radiation and exposure to it is about, I suggest studying the excellent graphic below produced by the Uranium Information Center that the World Health Organization uses, which will help you realize what's involved in the high and low ends of the energy spectrum.

Looking closely, you will note that *Cosmic, Gamma, and X-Ray* radiation are classified as *Ionising* [sic] *Radiation.* Gamma and X-ray are what we would call "man-made technology" radiation.

World Health Organization & Uranium Information Center

World Health Organization & Uranium Information Center[56]

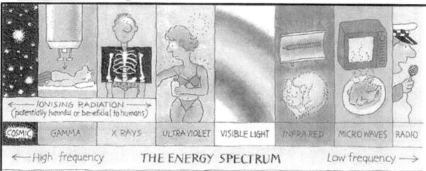

Cosmic ionizing radiation is out in space and one of the reasons astronauts must use space suits for protection. The solar wind, which contains cosmic radiation, can cause much mischief with satellites and electronics. The earth's magnetic field is in constant battle with radiation from *solar radionoise* storms. Sometimes there are *geomagnetic* storms that can knock out power grids on earth and affect the *aurorae borealis*—the Northern and Southern Lights around the poles. There is nothing we can do about that. What we can control is our exposure to man-made ionizing radiation.

Check out where microwaves either from cell phones or ovens come in on the energy spectrum: *low frequency radiation*, sometimes referred to as ELFs, extremely low frequencies.

Medical Ionizing Radiation

Mammograms

There's something that I don't understand quite frankly, and I'd like to see if my readers think that there is some sort of anomaly between what's said about safety and the push in promoting annual mammograms and what an online *New York Times* article titled "Breast Cancer" in the October 18, 2011, issue said:

> ***Radiation*** *– If you received radiation therapy as a child or young adult to treat cancer of the chest area, you have a much higher risk for developing breast cancer. The younger you started such radiation and the higher the dose, the higher your risk – especially if the radiation was given during breast development.* [57]

According to the National Cancer Institute,

> ***Radiation*** *exposure—Mammograms require very small doses of radiation. The risk of harm from this radiation exposure is low, but repeated x-rays have the potential to cause cancer. The benefits, however, nearly always outweigh the risk.* [58]

Cumulative ionizing radiation that a 45-year-old woman would have received as a result of mammograms could be up to 24 mSv. [59]

Consider how many mammograms a woman receives at the encouragement of breast cancer advocacy groups and the amount of ionizing radiation pumped into breast tissue. Something doesn't seem to comport science-wise, I think. Mull over the fact that most women have more than one X-ray exposure during mammography. Ouch!

December 2, 2009 *Medscape* published the article "Radiation Exposure From Annual Mammography Increases Breast Cancer Risk in Young High-Risk Women" wherein Fran Lowry reported on new research presented at the 95th Scientific Assembly of the Radiological Society of North America:

> *The low doses of radiation associated with annual screening mammography could be placing high-risk women in even more jeopardy of developing breast cancer, particularly if they start screening at a young age or have frequent exposure.* [59]

CT Scans

CT scans (computerized tomography) are not as benign as one assumes. According to an *Archives of Internal Medicine*, December 2009 article, "Radiation Dose Associated With Common Computed Tomography Examinations and the Associated Lifetime Attributable Risk of Cancer" an estimated 29,000 future cancers or malignancies could occur from the CT scans performed during 2007 alone. CT scans produce gamma rays, a form of ionizing radiation. The authors concluded,

> *Radiation doses from commonly performed diagnostic CT examinations are higher and more variable than generally quoted, highlighting the need for greater standardization across institutions.* [60]

According to *Absolute Astronomy's* website on **Ionizing Radiation**,

> …*damage done by ionizing radiation produces free radicals, even at room temperatures and below, and production of such free radicals is the reason these and other ionizing radiations produce quite different types of chemical effects from (low-temperature) heating. Free radical production is also a primary basis for the particular danger to biological systems of relatively small amounts of ionizing radiation that are far smaller than needed to produce significant heating. Free radicals easily damage DNA, and ionizing radiation may also directly damage DNA by ionizing or breaking DNA molecules. … Exposure to radiation causes damage to living tissue, and can result in mutation, radiation sickness, cancer, and death.* [61]

Unfortunately, medicine uses too many ionizing radiation-producing diagnostic procedures and treatments in the management of cancer and other diseases, I think. Ionizing radiation scares the living daylights out of anyone who knows the damage it can cause. That reason alone should be one of OSHA's concerns for airport screeners working with the TSA's ionizing radiation X-ray machines that airline passengers must walk through. TSA workers are constantly bombarded and being exposed from working in such close proximity to the TSA's X-ray backscatter machines.

Radiation Treatments

More than half of the patients with cancer are treated with radiation therapy that supposedly kills cancer cells and shrinks tumors. During such treatment, one also can receive burns and acquire radiation sickness from exposure. There are various side effects to radiation treatment, including losing one's hair. Fatigue can last for as long as six weeks after treatments.

One of the dangers of radiation treatment is discussed in the paper "Risk of second malignancies after adjuvant radiotherapy for breast cancer: a large-scale, single-institution review" published in 2007 that concluded,

> *Although radiation therapy (RT) has been shown to reduce 15-year mortality in breast cancer, it is associated with an increased risk of some types of secondary malignancy.* [62]

The Lancet published an article in its November 30, 1974 issue that was not favorable to irradiation therapy when compared with women treated by mastectomy only. Although that was back in 1974, it may be something to think about and consider. The results

> *Of controlled clinical trials so far published, all six, including more than 3400 patients, decreased survival of between 1 and 10% in irradiated patients when compared with those treated by mastectomy alone.* [63]

Radiation sickness often is coupled with adverse effects from chemotherapy, which can be everything from:

- Low white blood cell count (myleosuppressive; febrile neutropenia)
- ***Plus 198 other side effects*** listed on *ChemoCare.com* that include anything alphabetically from *Abdominal pain* to *Xerostomia.* 64

Note: If you have sickle cell anemia, make certain you tell your physicians that *before you start any type of chemotherapy.*

According to some patients, who opted out of 'gold stand-ard' treatments and then went the holistic route, treatments often bordered on torment, were debilitating, and some claimed agonizing.

Moreover, allopathic cancer management patients often must take several rounds of chemotherapy and go through numerous and sundry adverse side effects time after time.

Are you aware that a survey done by *The Los Angeles Times* and the McGill Cancer Center, Montreal, Canada, exposed the shocking fact that 75 to 91 percent of oncologists—the very doctors who prescribe and administer chemotherapy to cancer patients—would *refuse* chemotherapy if they were faced with cancer? Perhaps they are aware that chemotherapy is effective with only 2 to 4 percent of cancers, according to Ralph Moss, PhD, cancer patient advocate and author of the book, *Questioning Chemotherapy.*

One of the most frightening adverse effects of chemo-therapy that most cancer patients are not told about is what is referred to as "chemobrain." The *Journal of the National Cancer Institute* published the article "Chemobrain is Real but

May Need New Name" January 29, 2009 wherein the author candidly spoke of *"the nearly ubiquitous experience of foggy thinking immediately after chemotherapy treatment..."* [65] That, more than anything, was something I did not want to experience—losing my absolutely sharp brain and memory for me would be a disaster, as I'm a researcher and writer.

There are other published articles about brain fog and memory loss with breast cancer treatment that you may want to check out:

- "Cognitive functioning of postmenopausal breast cancer patients before adjuvant systemic therapy, and its association with medical and psychological factors" [66]
- "Effects of Tamoxifen and Exemestane on Cognitive Functioning of Postmenopausal Patients With Breast Cancer: Results From the Neuropsychological Side Study of the Tamoxifen and Exemestane Adjuvant Multinational Trial" [67]

The Institute of Science in Society (ISIS) website <i-sis.org.uk/FO12.php> discusses topics that cancer patients need to consider seriously: electronic fields doubling leukemia rates, microwaves, and mobile (cell) phones. The information is not meant to scare you. However, many scientists agree it is prudent to avoid and/or limit exposure to such radiation. If you are a person who spends driving time with a cell phone hooked up to your ear, you just may want to take seriously the information discussed. I think it can help you better understand some dynamics involved that you may not know about and also increase your ability to defeat breast cancer.

For information about electromagnetic radiation from cell phones, computers, etc., please visit this informative web site <electricsense.com/1326/how-to-evaluate-your-level-of-elec-tromagnetic-radiation-exposure/>. In the left side menu *Latest Articles*, I think you may be interested in "Electrosensitivity – Healing and Treatment."

Want a natural cosmetic to brighten up a face?
Brush on a smile.

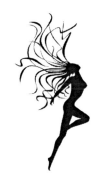

Chapter Ten

Chemotherapy and Renal Failure

Many physicians who clearly see a fact they cannot explain simply deny that it exists.

… Galen the Physician (CE 129—199)
Roman-Greek physician, surgeon & philosopher

Dr Suzanne Humphries, MD, *nephrologist*, states that patients undergoing chemotherapy often experience renal failure:

> *BK polyoma is also a recognized complication of kidney failure in patients undergoing immunosuppression for cancers and for non-renal organ transplants.[44]While BK polyoma is considered a rare complication, renal failure is not rare in patients undergoing chemotherapy. Without a more comprehensive investigation in the area of renal failure during chemotherapy, it will remain unknown how often these problems are silently occurring. Most cases of renal failure during chemotherapy are simply called tubular necrosis and are not deeply investigated.* [68]

How sad and totally disturbing that damaging side effects to the kidneys occur during chemotherapy. It appears that only palliative treatment may be given for renal failure. Or, is that when oncologists decide a cancer patient has to get his or her affairs in order?

One would think that preventing renal failure would be of paramount concern during cancer treatment, since the kidneys are 'prime time' organs for 'toxic waste disposal' via the urinary tract.

To understand better Dr Humphries comments and concerns, you may want to read her extraordinary paper "Vaccination and Renal Patients: A critical examination of assumed safety and effectiveness," October 4, 2011, published by the *International Medical Council on Vaccinations* at <vaccinationcouncil.org/2011/10/04/suzanne-humphries-md-medical-doctor-vaccination-risks-renal-patients-kidneys/>.

Dr Humphries is a practicing MD (nephrologist) and homeopath who understands how kidneys are designed to function by Nature. As such, she has seen professionally the damage done to kidneys by heavy duty, toxic chemotherapy cancer treatment drugs. To learn more about Dr Humphries and her medical practice, you may want to visit her web site < http://drsuzanne.net/about/>.

When in doubt, check it out thoroughly.

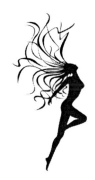

Chapter Eleven
Mammograms: The Supposed 'Gold Standard' for Breast Cancer Diagnosis

You start out happy that you have no hips or boobs.
All of a sudden you get them, and it feels sloppy.
Then just when you start liking them, they start drooping.

… Cindy Crawford (1966—)
Supermodel & Designer

Certainly every female remembers when she began to flower and develop breasts. With that came one of the frills of womanhood, wearing a bra. Can you remember how excited you were when your mom took you shopping for your very first bra? Little did we realize then that with breasts would come monthly self-breast examinations and, as we grew older, especially since 1983 when mammograms became widespread, prodding by the medical establishment for annual mammograms. But did any of us ever question the safety and efficacy of mammograms?

Regardless of what mammogram advocates say, there really is a downside with serious repercussions to mammograms. One downside was calibration of the X-ray equipment, which, hopefully, has been corrected. Numerous peer-reviewed studies have been published about mammography screening, which I think women, and my readers in particular, ought to know about because those studies are not shared with women in most instances. What women only hear is, "Mammograms save lives." Let's review what scientific articles say about mammograms.

In the November 24, 2008 issue of the *Archives of Internal Medicine*, researchers PH Azhl, J Maehlen, and HG Welch published, "The natural history of invasive breast cancers detected by screening mammography" wherein they state that invasive breast cancers were 22 percent HIGHER in women who had mammograms over a five year period in Norway than women who did not have regular mammograms.

Another article, "Incidence of and treatment for ductal carcinoma in situ of the breast," published in *JAMA* in March 1996 stated that *ductal carcinoma in situ* has increased 328 percent since the widespread screening use of mammograms began in 1983.

Dr Samuel Epstein, MD, stated in his 2001 article, "Dangers and Unreliability of Mammography: Breast Examination is a Safe, Effective, and Practical Alternative," that mammograms carry many dangers, including the *"induction and promotion of breast cancer."* Dr Epstein came to that conclusion after reviewing 47 scientific articles on mammograms at the Chicago School of Public Health.

Then there are false positives that come with mammography. [69] As high as 70 to 80 percent of positive mammograms are false positives, as proven either by needle or surgical biopsy. Another problem with mammography is women who have dense breasts that the mammogram cannot 'read' correctly. For women with dense breasts or breast implants, mammograms basically are useless and only pump ionizing radiation into breast tissue and the body.

Probably a much more reliable confirmation of a tumor would be an ultrasound that uses sound waves to make a picture (sonogram) of the breast tissue. Ultrasound can detect something a mammogram has difficulty doing or cannot do and that is 'see' and 'picture' the breast tissue next to the chest wall. Ultrasound can tell if the lump is filled with fluid—a cyst—or if it is a solid lump, a tumor.

However, there is a much more reliable diagnostic test for breast cancer; it's thermography which photographs the patterns of heat waves that are generated by cancer cells in breast tissue. Any area where there is abnormal cell growth produces extra heat that then is captured and photographed by thermography. See Chapter 45 *Thermography* for more detailed information. Thermography is what I chose rather than expose my breasts and lungs to ionizing radiation from mammograms.

The Lancet published an article in 1995, "Screening mammography and public health policy: the need for perspective" by C Wright and C Mueller wherein they stated something very profound, I think:

Assessment of benefit is contentious, but assessment of harm caused by mammography is direct and simple: false-positives cause unnecessary interventions; false negatives give inappropriate reassurance. There are false hopes and expectations of cure, high levels of public fear and anxiety about breast cancer, radiation hazards, and diversion of massive healthcare resources. …

For public health policy decisions about allocation of resources for breast screening, one needs a measure of added years of life (or "lives saved") rather than lives "at risk" after diagnosis. …

In view of what we know about the cytokinetics of the disease, we should not be surprised that the eventual outcome (death due to breast cancer) for the large majority of women is unaffected by screening mammography. The growth rates of breast cancers are highly variable, but in most cases the disease has been present for many years before it is diagnosable by any means. About 40 doublings of breast cancer cells create a lethal tumour [sic] burden, yet mammography cannot detect a mass until 25-30 doublings have already occurred. [70]

I disagree totally with *"before it is diagnosable by any means."* Thermography can and does diagnose "hot" abnormal cancer cell growth extremely early in the process of cell division.

There's a newer, more advanced mammogram, the CAD (computer-aided detection) that supposedly helps radiologists get a better read on mammograms, which, by the way, probably is the primary cause for more false positive readings. So why does the medical profession and cancer advocacy groups still promote mammograms?

Mammograms supposedly are the 'tried and true' first line of diagnostics when it comes to screening for breast cancer. Numerous studies indicate various conclusions, however, the paper "Effect of mammography screening on surgical treatment for breast cancer in Norway: comparative analysis of cancer registry data" published in the *British Medical Journal* September 13, 2011 *about the effects of mammograms,* I think, says something about that screening process, i.e., over-diagnosis.

> **Conclusions** *Mammography screening in Norway was associated with a noticeable increase in rates for breast cancer surgery in women aged 50-69 (the age group invited to screening) and also an increase in mastectomy rates.* **Although over-diagnosis is likely to have caused the initial increase in mastectomy rates and the overall increase in surgery rates in the age group screened,** *the more recent decline in mastectomy rates has affected all age groups and is likely to have resulted from changes in surgical policy.* [71]
> [CJF emphasis added]

Mastectomy and overall increase in surgery rates are most unfortunate, in my opinion.

In the *Discussion* section of the above paper, we find that

> *A potential benefit of mammography screening—a reduction in mastectomy rates and an increase the use of less invasive surgery—was not corroborated by our results, which show that mastectomy rates in Norway have declined similarly in invited and non-invited age groups from the pre-screening period (1993-5) to the more recent screening period (2005-8). ...*
>
> *During the introduction of screening, mastectomy rates in invited women aged 50-69 increased by 9%. In contrast, during the same period the rates in non-invited women decreased by 17% in the 40-49 age group and by 13% in the 70-79 age group. This corresponds to a 31% increase in the relative risk of mastectomy in women invited to screening compared with the non-invited younger age group. Mastectomy rates noticeably increased in Akershus, Oslo, Rogaland, and Hordaland counties when screening started in 1996. ...*
>
> *The mastectomy rates for stages 0, I, and II increased in women aged 50-69 in the first years of the screening introduction phase. Rates decreased for all stages except III and IV from 2002-3, reflecting that changes in surgical practice affect both lymph node positive and negative invasive cancers with a diameter less than 5 cm, as well as ductal carcinoma in situ. Rates of breast surgery have increased especially for stages 0 and I, but also for stage II. ...*[71]

If an increase in mastectomy rates occurred in Norway, we can only imagine what is going on in the United States, where a large medical sub-culture has sprung up within women's breast cancer issues, i.e., reconstructive breast surgery.

According to *Wikipedia,*

> *The mastectomy rate was highest in central and eastern Europe at 77%. The USA had the second highest rate of mastectomy with 56%, western and northern Europe averaged 46%, southern Europe 42% and Australia and New Zealand 34%.*[72]

We must not forget to consider that male breast cancer patients also receive mastectomies.

According to the National Breast Cancer Coalition *Facts and Statistics about Breast Cancer in the United States – 2011,*

> *Mammography screening does not prevent or cure breast cancer. It may detect the disease before symptoms occur. It may also lead to over diagnosis and over treatment (Nelson et al, 2009).*
>
> *Mammography screening has led to a dramatic increase in the incidence of ductal carcinoma in situ (DCIS). The diagnosis was relatively rare before the early 1980's and the widespread use of mammography. Today, approximately one woman is diagnosed with DCIS for every four women diagnosed with invasive breast cancer (Allegra et al, 2010).*[73]

Something I need to mention, I think, is that even though breast cancer in women under 25 years of age is considered rare, it seems to be on the increase. Perhaps birth control pills, which play around with female hormones that are taken to be safe from becoming pregnant while being sexually active, just may be *part* of what is upping the rate of breast cancers in *young* women. Therefore, the need for women of all ages— particularly young women—to understand the apparent varied dynamics that play parts in female breast cancer besides genetics, which statistically counts for between 5 and 10 percent only. [74]

The website <breastcancer.org/risk/factors/genetics.jsp> has within it a link to BRCA 1 and BRCA 2 genetic testing, which may be of interest to those who want to go that route. However and personally, *I think* the best and more accurate route for a prophylactic diagnostic approach would be blood tests (CA15-3 and CA 27-29) that could be taken every six months and thermography—annually if need be—which does not put ionizing radiation into the body, yet picks up very early cancer cells because of the heat they generate that is photographically captured and registered by thermography.

A Change in Prophylactic Breast Cancer Diagnostic Practices
The medical profession is having second thoughts about mammograms—to some extent—and may be coming around to a more *holistic* way of thinking, although not totally, which I hope would be to use thermography/thermograms that don't discharge ionizing radiation into the breast and body.

In 2009 the U.S. Preventive Services Task Force said that annual mammograms to check for breast cancer are needed only every other year starting at age 50. However, the American Cancer Society and women's breast cancer advocacy groups still advise annual mammograms starting at age 40.

In October 2011, a large study found there were more false alarms, i.e., false positives, for women who got annual mammograms than those who opted to receive them every other year. Dr Michael LeFevre, one of the USPS Task Force members and a professor of family and community medicine at the University of Missouri, said, *"The more tests that you do, the more likely you are to be faced with a false-positive test,"* which leads to unnecessary biopsies and possible harm. I could not agree more with Dr LeFevre's assessment since, in my opinion, the more stress factors upon delicate breast tissue—biopsies and surgeries are stresses—the more cells are likely to become damaged either from procedures or chemicals used to sedate, biopsy, and/or treat.

Do Annual Mammograms Lead to Secondary Cancers?

Since I started on this odyssey with my right breast, I've met numerous people with various types of cancers in holistic healthcare therapy rooms where horror stories about conventional cancer treatments rival campfire ghost stories that are told, only none of their stories are funny in any way.

I'd like to share the story of a lovely professional lady who told me her sad story about thyroid cancer that she finally sought holistic medical care in treating. When she found out

I was writing this book, she wanted to talk. Her first question to me was about mammograms. It seemed all of a sudden during our conversation she experienced an aha moment. I could see a light bulb go on in her mind when she sheepishly admitted, "I've had annual mammograms since I was 20, and now I'm 49 and have thyroid cancer. Is there any connection, do you think?"

She and I discussed the procedures in taking breast screening X-rays; how many repeat shots/exposures on an annual visit; and that there's ionizing radiation that was shot into her body every time and in close proximity to the thyroid/parathyroid in the upper chest area. Coincidentally, one of the contributing factors for breast cancer is chest X-rays or X-ray treatment for other health problems of the chest.

Her immediate retort was that she was scheduled to have a mammogram on the advice of her gynecologist and was putting it off because of all the CTs and MRIs she had recently in diagnosing the thyroid cancer. Is there anything that I would recommend, she asked? I told her that I had thermography, an FDA-approved diagnostic procedure that did not involve any type of radiation, particularly ionizing radiation from X-rays. She could not thank me enough for telling her about thermography. However, she did have a subsequent mammogram I learned. When I asked why because I thought she was going to have a thermogram instead, she said her gynecologist prevailed upon her. Need I say more!

I relate this true story because there's more than a probability that her thyroid cancer could have been a secondary cancer caused by ionizing radiation from diagnostic procedures. To illustrate radiologically what I contend, please consider this from *Nuclear Chemistry The Biological Effects of Nuclear Radiation* by Dr Frank Settle:

> *When radiation strikes complex biological molecules, such as proteins or nucleic acids, it may fracture the molecules and prevent their proper functioning. This can result in loss of cell vitality, decreased enzyme activity, **initiation of cancer, and genetic mutations.** The immediate effects of acute exposure to radiation are caused by free radicals rupturing the cell membranes. This rupturing causes the cells to lose their contents and die. If enough cells are killed, functions associated with the cells cease. Death occurs because of the direct loss of vital organs or because of secondary infections resulting from the breakdown of the immune system. The effect depends on the dose of radiation received.* [75]
> [CJF emphasis added]

That's another reason I elected to go the holistic route, and not risk direct loss of vital organs, or infections resulting from the breakdown of the immune system, or a secondary cancer. Everything done in holistic cancer treatments is to **support and build up** the immune system to defeat and conquer cancer, plus I won't lose my hair or suffer radiation burns to my chest.

The *Journal of the National Cancer Institute* published the article "Estimated risk of radiation-induced breast cancer from mammographic screening for young BRCA mutation carriers" February 4, 2009 wherein that very issue was discussed. Furthermore, it is estimated that as high as 80 percent of all positive mammograms really are false positives, which require biopsies to prove there is cancer. However, if there is cancer, then the biopsy has the capability of spreading cancer cells. That was documented in the paper "Manipulation of the primary breast tumor and the incidence of sentinel node metastases from invasive breast cancer" published in the *Archives of Surgery,* June 2004. [76]

Ultrasounds (sonograms) are proving more accurate than mammograms in the detection of breast cancer. That's documented in "Increasing accuracy of detection of breast cancer with 3-T MRI" in the *American Journal of Roentgenology,* April 2009.

One of the more sophisticated diagnostics for breast cancer is MR-Spectroscopy, which is an alternative to biopsy. It can detect cancer from the choline peak in tumor cells. The procedure has been discussed in the article "Proton MR Spectroscopy with Choline Peak as Malignancy Marker Improves Positive Predictive Value for Breast Cancer Diagnosis: Preliminary Study" in the 2006 issue of *Radiology.* [77] In another article, MRS using choline was reported as accurately having evaluated patients with *recurrent* breast cancer masses *after* breast cancer treatment and radiation therapy.

As I write this chapter a dustup about mammograms is occurring in Great Britain and it's looking like a boxing match may have just begun. Both sides of the issue are putting on 'the gloves' for what may be an ugly match. In September 2011 researchers at the Nordic Cochrane Centre in Denmark made claims that the British National Health Services (NHS) breast cancer screening was misinforming women who had mammograms. What? How? Well, women were not told the harms of over diagnosis, which far outweigh the benefits, was the complaint.

Professor Susan Bewley, a consultant obstetrician at King's College, published an open letter in the *British Medical Journal* addressed to Sir Mike Richards, national cancer director at the Department of Health, wherein she said she found NHS leaflets *"exaggerated benefits and did not spell out the risks. … The oft-repeated statement that '1,400 lives a year are saved' has not been subjected to proper scrutiny. Even cancer charities use lower estimates."* Sir Richards responded with, *"I will do my best to achieve consensus on the evidence, though I realise* [sic] *this may not ultimately be possible."* To which this author says, "Consensus! What consensus?" Does that mean that radiologists will have more input and say about ionizing radiation going into women's breasts via mammography? I think I can predict the outcome even before any consensus is ever proclaimed. It will be the same old, same old, "Mammograms save lives."

But there are other aspects to the problem. How many lives do mammograms *doom* to secondary cancers? How many diagnoses *do mammograms miss*? How many *false positives* do they find that necessitate biopsies? Perhaps there is too much of a profitable industry built around mammograms that apparently veils the facts. In my opinion, it's a shame, if not a tragedy, that women don't know what's really going on. I do, and that's why I chose the holistic approach for me.

"Every day in every way, I'm getting better"
should be our mantra.

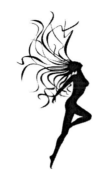

Chapter Twelve

Let's Talk Mammograms Again

The hardest years in life are those between ten and seventy.

… Helen Hayes (1900—1993)
American actress quoted at age 73

*T*his chapter may sound repetitious, but I think it is appropriate that I explain as clearly as possible information that women have not been told and can make a difference in breast cancer statistics both for diagnoses and survival rates.

Please reconsider this information:

> **Conclusions** *Mammography screening in Norway was associated with a noticeable increase in rates for breast cancer surgery in women aged 50-69 (the age group invited to screening) and also an increase in mastectomy rates.* **Although over-diagnosis is likely to have caused the initial increase in mastectomy rates and the overall increase in surgery rates in the age group screened,** *the*

more recent decline in mastectomy rates has affected all age groups and is likely to have resulted from changes in surgical policy. [78] [CJF emphasis added]

And again, according to *Wikipedia,*

The mastectomy rate was highest in central and eastern Europe at 77%. The USA had the second highest rate of mastectomy with 56%, western and northern Europe averaged 46%, southern Europe 42% and Australia and New Zealand 34%. [79]

It's important to note and not forget that male breast cancer patients also receive mastectomies. Years ago I was consulted on diet by a gentleman who had had male breast cancer surgery, and he was distraught because no one was able to tell him what to do about the diet-cancer connection. That was in the early 1980s when the diet-disease connection was considered quackery by MDs and RDs alike. Boy, have they had their hats turned around since then. Nevertheless, in my opinion, they still are not where they need to be, since they have not exposed GMO, chemically grown, and processed foods for nutritional polemics plus the health dangers scientific studies confirm, which certainly are not in the best health interests nor nutritional status of anyone, especially women with breast cancer.

In Chapter 11 I introduced, "According to the National Breast Cancer Coalition *Facts and Statistics about Breast Cancer in the United States – 2011,*

Mammography screening does not prevent or cure breast cancer. It may detect the disease before symptoms occur. It may also lead to over diagnosis and over treatment (Nelson et al, 2009).

Mammography screening has led to a dramatic increase in the incidence of ductal carcinoma in situ (DCIS). The diagnosis was relatively rare before the early 1980's and the widespread use of mammography. Today, approximately one woman is diagnosed with DCIS for every four women diagnosed with invasive breast cancer (Allegra et al, 2010). [80]

Something I think I need to mention again is that even though breast cancer in women under 25 years of age is considered rare, *it seems to be on the increase.* Perhaps birth control pills, which play around with female hormones and are taken to be safe from becoming pregnant while being sexually active, just may be *part* of what is upping the rate of breast cancers in young women. Think hormones and cancer! Therefore, there's the need for women of all ages—particularly young women—to understand the apparent varied dynamics that take part in female breast cancer besides genetics, which statistically accounts for only between 5 and 10 percent. [81]

BreastCancer.org at <breastcancer.org/risk/factors/genetics.jsp> had embedded in it a link to BRCA 1 and BRCA 2 genetic testing [81], which may be of interest to those who want to go that route. However and personally, I think a better and more accurate route or prophylactic approach for those who feel genetics may be involved would be blood tests (CA

15-3 and CA 27-29), which could be taken every six months. Additionally, annual or biennial thermography, which does not put ionizing radiation into the body but picks up *very early* cancer cells due to the heat they put out that is 'seen' by thermography and transformed into visible color photographs.

Are There Dangers to Mammograms?

Have you ever asked that question? Perhaps after reading this, you may think twice about what you hear regarding annual mammograms. In 2011 the American College of Obstetricians and Gynecologists released a set of new guidelines for mammograms encouraging more women to get mammograms starting at an earlier age, which radiologists also recommend. What would you expect? They certainly aren't going to not recommend them.

To corroborate that mammograms do not reduce the number of deaths from breast cancer, the *British Medical Journal* published an article regarding just that. Dr Otis Brawley, MD, chief medical officer for the American Cancer Society, made this statement, which I think shows some introspection on his part, particularly in the parts that I've highlighted:

> *The American Cancer Society continues to advise women age forty and older to get a high quality mammogram and clinical breast examination on a regular basis. … Women should know how their breasts normally look and feel, be alert for changes, and **when there are changes, seek expert help. Mammography is not perfect. It will not***

***detect all breast cancers, and not all women are at
an age when mammography is recommended. That's
why a heightened sense of awareness is an important
complement to regular mammography screening.*** [82]
[CJF emphasis added]

With all that's promoted about mammography being a life-saving diagnostic, one readily can realize how mammography also can be a dud either because of not picking up tumors, false positives, and ionizing radiation, which can induce secondary cancers in the body. Mammography's 'state of the art' *computer-aided-detection* (CAD) software technique is touted as helping radiologists better-read mammograms. Would you like to know some of the statistics about CAD?

The *Journal of the National Cancer Institute* published a study July 27, 2011 wherein the study's author Dr Joshua A Fenton said this:

> *''All in all, we found very little impact of CAD on the out-comes of mammography.''* [83]

That study was based on 1.6 million screening mammograms in seven states from 1998 to 2006. Furthermore, Dr Fenton added:

> *For every 200 women who are screened with CAD who have a second mammogram, one additional woman is called back unnecessarily for further testing.* [83]

To which I would like to add, additional ionizing radiation that *is cumulative* in the body and can lead to secondary cancers. Guess what? CAD also adds about twelve additional dollars to the cost of a mammogram. *Caching!* To 'guild the lily', in my opinion, the American College of Radiology states that CAD *"may slightly increase the sensitivity of mammographic interpretations."* And here's the catcher, I think: CAD may be the cause or the link to an increase of recalled patients, many of which are not necessary, to receive additional mammographic exposures. So what does that say and possibly prove?

Why may it seem as if I'm coming down on mammograms, a supposed life-saving diagnostic for women? Because there is something women can do that is much more safe, accurate, and effective in prophylactic diagnostic care, and that is thermography which 'sees' cancer cell 'hot spots' very early in cancer, along with blood tests that can be taken every six months for those who consider themselves at higher risks for breast cancer. See Chapter 34, *Holistic Preventive Measures* for more information.

Lastly, you may want to consider what was published in the *Archives of Internal Medicine* October 24, 2011 in an article that concluded,

> *Most women with screen-detected breast cancer have not had their life saved by screening. They are instead either diagnosed early (with no effect on their mortality) or over-diagnosed.* [84]

Ouch! Is what I have to say. But then, the article authors are just being candid. Additionally, the article went on to say that for all age groups, life-saving mammography screening was less than 25 percent. Now, since you know such information about mammograms, maybe doing something different will find breast cancer much earlier. May I suggest a thermogram, at least to get a base line reading, and as part of your annual physical, have cancer/tumor marker blood tests drawn, which are discussed in Chapter 34 *Holistic Preventive Measures To Avoid Breast Cancer*.

There's always another or better way of doing anything.

Part II

Holistic Non-Toxic BREAST Cancer SELF-Management

Following the *'Manufacturer's Manual'* That Comes With the Human Body

And God said, Behold, I have given you every herb bearing seed, which is on the face of all the earth, and every tree, in the which is the fruit of a tree yielding seed; to you it shall be for meat.

Genesis 1:29 KJV

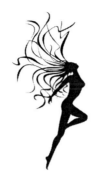

Chapter Thirteen
Empowering YOURSELF to Wellness

*You may never know what results come of your action,
but if you do nothing there will be no result.*

... **Mahatma Gandhi (1869—1948)**
Political & Ideological leader of India

*Authentic empowerment is the knowing that you are on purpose,
doing God's work, peacefully and harmoniously.*

... **Wayne Dyer, PhD (1940—)**
Motivational speaker and Author

*F*rom my viewpoint the most important and powerful action you can take immediately—if not sooner—is to believe in yourself and the power within you to overcome your problem to be well again, regardless of what frightening statistics you may read or hear, whatever well-intended medical professionals may tell you, or any personal fears and doubts you may have.

Please stop and read that again, then think about what that sentence really is saying. Close your eyes for a minute and let its message seep into your being and become a part of you because that resolve will be what will get you through your therapy, no matter which route you chose to go. When we believe, it will happen—it will. Isn't there a saying that goes something like, "When I believe it, I will see it"? Sounds strange—even esoteric—but the power of the energy in the mind truly works that way.

Now—probably more than any time in your life—is when you have to realize, understand, and accept that your mind is more powerful than you probably thought or knew it to be. Some say we use only ten percent of our brain. However, the mind is a totally different 'animal' or entity from the organ we call brain. Our mind is consciousness or the mainframe computer of our lives. It's what we are about and part of what makes us, us or what some call our spirit or soul. Consciousness is what travels with us before, during, and after our earthly encounter. It's energy and energy transforms; it cannot die. Don't believe that? Check out this remarkable video <disclose.tv/action/viewvideo/51274/ Spiritual_Reality__Near_Death_Experiences__2010_/> wherein folks relate their near death experiences; what they remember vividly; and apparent reasons why they are still alive. They learned the lessons of love, trust, and fulfillment, which are very freeing.

After you experience the 'shock of your life' or whatever you may want to call a diagnosis of breast cancer, you seriously have to get down to the business of taking responsibility for getting well. In addition to all the therapies, lifestyle, and dietary changes you ought to be making, you will come to realize just how important it is to have your head on straight about what you are facing.

May I remind you that stress has to be eliminated from your life because studies have found that those who are prone to stress are more likely to develop breast cancer. Please read that last sentence again, then stop and ponder how much stress is in your life and what you are going to do to eliminate it. That's something that must be taken on very early in the game of cheating and beating breast cancer.

Nothing helps to get to that enduring place like meditation and prayer, I truly believe. I can hear you saying, "Oh, here she goes on a soapbox," or "She's gonna preach about some religion." No, I definitely will do neither. What I will do is ask you to go within yourself and find *the* spiritual route *you* want to take to contact your higher self [consciousness, spirit energy, soul] and make the resolve to work a *spiritual exercise* daily—even several times a day if that's what it takes to get you over the hump—to believe in yourself, and fight the good fight to wellness.

Some may opt for meditation—I do that as part of my prayer routine—first thing every morning upon awakening. I can spend anywhere from thirty to ninety minutes depending upon how involved I become.

May I share with you my perceived difference between prayer and meditation? I believe prayer is my talking with the Higher Being, Creator God; meditation is my listening to Creator God talking with me. It can and does happen. We need no go-betweens; it's all there right inside our consciousness. Within each and every one of us is an energy source that not only makes life possible, but also enables us to be who we are. We are part of a dynamic energy force—Creation—that in recent years has become fashionable to deny.

Once you become addicted to meditation and/or prayer, you won't be able to go without its uplifting, affirming, and transformational fruits or gifts of acceptance and peace. Those gifts are so powerfully helpful in making our way through these trying times that I cannot encourage you enough to consider going within to find your *key* to unlocking the door to peace and well being.

For those who may be inquisitive as to how I start my meditation, may I share the opening prayer?

I place the radiant White Light of God,
The Gold Light of God's Love,
The Violet Flame of Transformation,
The Undifferentiated Light of Creator God,
And the Emerald Green Healing Ray of God
In, around, and through my Physical, Emotional, Mental, and
Spiritual Being.

However, I'm certain your creative thinking can come up with a beautiful greeting that will start you on your way to something you may not have considered to be a part of your treatment program: *prayer and meditation.* Please try it before you come to any conclusions about it. MRI brain scans document physical changes take place in our bodies when we meditate. It's been documented that the limbic system also gets activated to regulate relaxation.

WebMed online has an exceptional article "Can Prayer Heal? Does prayer have the power to heal? Scientists have some surprising answers" by Jeanie Lerche Davis that you may want to consider reading at <webmd.com/balance/features/can-prayer-heal>.

For readers who would like others to pray for you, there are numerous Internet prayer request sites where kind-hearted strangers gladly will pray for you. I've listed several to help you get started.

Prayer Request Websites

Grace Prayer Community, a Christian prayer site <graceprayer.org/?gclid=CPXs5Izhn6sCFQHf4Aodvgryiw>

The Franciscan Friars St. Anthony Shrine, a Catholic prayer site <stanthony.org/prayers/submit.asp>

A special note of interest for those of the Catholic faith.

The Catholic Church designated a special patron saint of cancer patients, St. Peregrine. You may want to visit a website in his honor, *St. Peregrine – Patron Saint of Cancer Patients* at <saintgeo.com/peregrine.htm>. There also is a link for prayer requests on that St. Peregrine website.

A Cancer Answer

Also, there's a biopharmaceutical company that develops and manufacturers monoclonal antibodies for the treatment of cancer and viral infections. Would you believe its name is *Peregrine Pharmaceuticals, Inc.*? I find that rather interesting or telling. What do you think?

Buddhists Beliefs about Prayer
<buddhanet.net/budsas/ebud/whatbudbeliev/198.thm>
Jewish Healing Prayer Request
<mhjconline.org/healingprayerrequest.htm>
Search for Prayers for Various Faiths
<beliefnet.com/Faiths/Prayer/Prayer-Search.aspx>

An Angel Prayer

Just about every religion and spiritual belief system acknowledges angels. Here's an angel prayer promoted by Tom T Moore in *The Gentle Way Book* that I'd like to share with my readers. Wanna know a secret? I say it daily.

Dear (Guardian) Angel, I ask for a most benevolent outcome for (mention your request) and may it be even better than I can hope for or expect. *Thank you.*

Before going further in this book regarding the most heart-wrenching health problem for an ever-growing number of females, may I ask that you please consider what's being offered about the need for a change of

138

paradigm relating to healthcare, which truly is nothing more than *perpetuated sickness care*, as this ten minute video accurately suggests <disclose.tv/action/viewvideo/21343/The_Living_Matrix__The_Science_of_Healing_Pt_8_8/>.

I hope and pray you find the peace of mind you seek, deserve, and treasure.

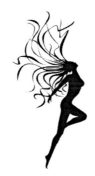

Chapter Fourteen

Importance of Nutrition in Managing Breast Cancer

The richness I achieve comes from nature, the source of my inspiration.

... Claude Monet (1840—1926)
French Impressionist artist

The significant and vital role that diet, *real food* nutrients, and nutrition play in the management and cure of any cancer—especially breast cancer—cannot be underestimated nor ignored. That's why my emphasis on it is so prominent in this book.

Think of it this way: Food—what we put into our bodies as nourishment—is the ages-old regimen we evolved with to provide fuel for bodies to function on all levels, e.g., micro—at cellular, and macro—as a human being. *Nothing changes body chemistry more than the food we put into it.*

Personally, I think our cars know more about fuel efficiency and performance than we do. Just imagine what would happen if you put sugar or water into your car's gas tank. Car engines were designed to run on petrol—not sugar or water—and now some run on ethanol blends, which seems to reduce the miles per gallon one gets from gasoline. At least that's what happens in my car: On ethanol-added gasoline, I get about 2 miles less to the gallon.

Human bodies are the ultimate in 'machinery'. They were built to run on real food, not chemicalized, denatured, or genetically modified foods. Those types of 'fuel' haven't been around as long as we have so when we eat them, they give us a 'kick', similar to what water in gasoline does in the gas tank in our cars.

The human body also can be considered as an extremely large test tube, since we add so many and varied chemicals from foods, edibles, nutrients, prescription drugs, municipal water systems, plus food manufacturing, animal and agricultural chemistry, that no one really knows the true interactions of possibly a thousand chemicals a day in the average modern diet and lifestyle. Stop and think about that.

Nevertheless, our bodies' cells do know—and react. The way they talk back to us about the inadequacies of *mal*nutrition is by using the language of disease. So, that's why cancer patients must change their diets to create both a hostile environment for cancer cells and an eco-friendly environment for the immune system to knock the stuffing out of cancer cells. Basically, it's that simple.

Keeping body chemistry at a proper pH and homeostasis, which holistic therapies are superb at doing I feel, means no heavy-duty toxic radiation or chemotherapy—at least for me. Even if a cancer patient subscribes to conventional allopathic cancer treatments, embarking on a course of holistic, *natural* nutrition and diet can make a significant impact and/or difference in quality of life while managing cancer utilizing allopathic cancer treatments.

If you remember, back in Chapter One I talked about the evolution of humans over time and how we interacted with Nature to get to where we are today without the technologies of the food processing and agricom industries. Most humans/families/communities grew their own food, survived, and thrived. Today 99 percent of the people in the United States do NOT grow their food, although many have summer gardens, which I truly believe is a godsend if gardeners are planting heirloom—not GMO—seeds and the soil is an alive and healthy growing medium. Therein is where nutrients and nutrition are found for growing food crops. That, however, is not the mechanism by which agricoms grow crops. They use chemical fertilizers, GMO seeds, plus pesticides and herbicides as if they were water.

All that chemicalization of food crops—especially fertilizers—affects not only nutrient uptake, but also impacts mineral content in the soil thereby making aluminum more available to crops, which they should not uptake. Big agra does not use sustainable agriculture methods such as planting green manure crops in the fall to winter over and then be turned under in spring to provide soil nutrients for growing food crops. That method is not cost effective to their way of doing business. Chemicalized farming methods produce nutrient deficient food crops and certainly less vital food for consumers, I do believe. Organic agriculture provides richer nutrients and higher nutritional values with no toxic chemical loads or residues.

Picture this. What would happen if you fed your pet goldfish, angelfish, or guppies crumbled up crackers or ground meat? *Don't do it, because they will die!* That's similar to what can happen when you feed the wrong kind of edibles to yourself and your family: cells in the body die—or mutate into cancer cells—from toxic chemicals and lack of nutrients. Pro-oxidants and free radicals in chemically grown foods are then utilized as 'nutrients' depriving cells of nutrition that induce cells to mutate.

That very fact about cellular nutrition is what molecular medicine doctors and holistic physicians understand without a doubt. That is why they restructure your diet to feed your body's cells into wellness, not chemicalize them further with chemotherapy and other toxins. Over and over during my practice as a *natural* nutritionist I used to tell clients, "You cannot poison a body into wellness." Man-made petrochemicals in the food supply and diet are not what Nature intended nor provided.

Diet, eating habits, food choices, cooking techniques, and anything revolving around the food you eat that does not contribute to it being nutrient-dense and as chemically-free as possible, will need to be changed *IF* you want to beat breast cancer, or any cancer. That's the key to changing body chemistry from crud to cure. Diet and nutrition are like magic genies in the cook pot and on a fork, so to speak. I know what I just said sounds a little off the wall, but if you don't take proper diet and nutrition seriously, you probably will not get the results you are hoping for.

Diet and nutrition are mainstays in the recipe for holistic wellness for any disease, especially breast cancer. May I give you an analogy to make my point? Think about your favorite recipe and what would happen if you omitted one or two of the main ingredients. You wouldn't have what you either had expected to make or were accustomed to tasting and eating. The same analogy applies to working on a holistic approach to curing cancer. It's a one-hundred-percent-plus commitment, I think.

From what I know, many women attest to their breast tumors literally disappearing without surgery, chemotherapy, or radiation after religiously staying with a raw foods and vegan/vegetarian—*and I add organically grown*—food diet. As I understand, Dr Nicholas Gonzalez's cancer patients, who do not have faulty protein digestion, and have solid breast tumors, confirm similar results. Dr Gonzalez's treatment prescribes a vegetarian/vegan diet consisting of fruits, vegetables, nuts, grains, and seeds—all organically grown, the same diet I've been following with the exception of adding an occasional organically grown egg. Furthermore, I've heard from numerous holistic physicians similar remarks, e.g., as long as breast cancer—or any cancer—patients stay on a vegetarian diet, tumors shrink away to nothing.

One last tidbit of dietary information I'd like to impress upon you is that cancer cells have more receptors for sugar than healthy normal cells. That is extremely important to know and remember, especially if your diet is high in starchy carbohydrates like breads, cakes, cereals—not whole grain—chips, cookies, crackers, donuts, pasta/spaghetti, pizza, popcorn, pop tarts, potatoes, pretzels, and white rice. Why? The reason is those edibles are converted into sugar during the digestive process that, in turn, feeds cancer cells and permits them to grow into tumors and/or metastasize. So you see how important diet is in the management of cancer and breast cancer, in particular. You don't want to feed cancer cells; you want to starve them while still feeding yourself.

I feel I must impress upon you that nothing—*nothing*—is going to impact body chemistry to combat breast cancer—or any type of cancer for that matter—as will the food you eat.

T Colin Campbell, PhD, published his findings linking poor nutrition as contributing to cancer in *The China Study: The Most Comprehensive Study of Nutrition Ever Conducted and the Startling Implications for Diet, Weight Loss, and Long-diagnosed cancers*. Interestingly, that study concluded that genetics accounts for only about 3 percent of cancers, while the remaining 97 percent was attributed to lifestyle factors, mainly food choices. May I suggest getting Dr Campbell's book to read?

Correct nutritious food intake is the only nutrient-providing element or modality you can get into the body three times a day that will effectuate change both as to the acid/

alkaline (pH) values and the nutritional and nutrient status for strengthening the immune system, plus helping to break down the outer mesh-like cell membrane of cancer cells. That almost impenetrable shell casing must be attacked and breached so that cancer cells can be killed off. Several agents can do that: chemotherapy, oxygen, hydrogen peroxide, and curcumin [turmeric], an Indian cooking spice that can induce cell apoptosis or cell 'suicide'.

Modified citrus pectin contains *galactosyl* residues, which are considered to be effective in hindering the spread of cancer cells. Here's some information on its effectiveness in the spread of cancer. Take special note of what it says about the surface of breast cancer cells.

> *Galactosyl residues can hinder the binding of carbohydrate-binding galectin 3, a type of protein commonly found on the surface of prostate,* **breast,** *brain, colon, skin, lymphatic, and larynx cells. Galectins are carbohydrate-binding proteins involved in the growth, survival, and spread (metastasis) of cancer, and they are present in abnormally high levels in many cancers.* [85] [CJF emphasis added]

Galactosyl pectin is not like the pectin a cook would use to make jellies and jams. It's an alkali soluble pectin powder supplement usually made from tomatoes. That's one of the reasons I used organically grown tomatoes with every meal, *galactosyl* residues. Then, there is fractionated pectin or modified citrus pectin, which is made from citrus, usually oranges.

Grapefruit pectin, however, needs a caveat because grapefruit juice has the ability to markedly elevate the bioavailability of prescription drugs. So please remember that important piece of information about galactosyl pectin.

Nutritious food nourishes the mind and also the soul.
Ever hear of soul food?

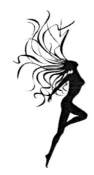

Chapter Fifteen
How the Body 'Interprets' Food

Worthless people live only to eat and drink;
people of worth eat and drink only to live.

… Socrates (469BCE—399BCE)
Greek Athenian philosopher

Do you recall my saying that the human body could be compared with the largest test tube? Well, now I'm going to give you an example of what I meant by that statement.

When we consume food, it must go through many digestive processes traveling the entire alimentary tract—about eight feet in length or 32 feet totally, if we include our intestines. During those travels body systems do a Herculean job of extracting nutrients and sending them on their way to the mitochondria in each and every cell—*except* cancer cells. They like sugar or foods that turn into sugar in the body for their 'nutrition'. This is where it's important to know about the *Glycemic Index* and how it comes into play.

One of the influentials affecting body chemistry is acid/alkaline balance or pH.

Food, when eaten, is treated by body chemistry processes that turn it into either an acid or alkaline ash. That, in turn, programs body chemistries into respective pH numbers. Some fluids are acid—the stomach, in particular, with its powerful hydrochloric acid—and others are alkaline, e.g., saliva. However, overall body pH should come in between 7.24 and 7.42—slightly alkaline—and no disease pattern, theoretically, should be able to set up shop, I learned.

It's been well established in holistic nutrition that more alkaline ash foods should be eaten than acid ash foods to influence a positive healing process within the body, no matter what the disease, but more so with cancer of any organ, especially breast cancer.

Acid Ash Forming Foods
American cheese
Artificial sweeteners
Aspirin
Bacon
Bagels
Beans and legumes
Beef
Beer (pH 2.5)
Black pepper
Black tea
Buffalo meat
Butter

Cheeses
Chicken
Chick peas/Garbanzo beans
Coffee (pH4)
Colas (pH 2)/Soft drinks
Condiments (most)
Cooking oils (all)
Corn syrup
Croissants
Eggs
Espresso
Fish
Hamburgers
Hard liquor and spirits
Ice cream
Lobster
Milk (both raw and pasteurized)
Milkshakes
Mussels
Quinoa
Red wine and white distilled vinegars
Saltine crackers
Sausage
Shrimp
Soybeans
Soymilk
Steak
Sugar, brown or white

Tobacco
Walnuts
White flour
Wine

Alkaline Ash Forming Foods
Almonds
Barley grass
Beets
Chestnuts
Coconut, fresh
Fermented vegetables
Garlic
Green juices
Millet
Most fruits *except* blueberries, cranberries, currants, plums, prunes
Most vegetables *except* corn, olives, winter squash
Mushrooms, including oriental varieties
Red chili pepper
Sea vegetables (seaweed)
Wheat grass

Regarding Food Allergies
It is important *NOT* to eat any foods to which you have food allergies, as doing that places strain on the immune system which, of course, you want to avoid since you are trying to build up the immune system.

Furthermore, I'd suggest not eating things you eat daily or crave.

Craving certain foods usually is an indication that your body is either hooked on or addicted to, or allergic to them, which could induce a possible weight gain factor, too.

You may experience withdrawal symptoms when you eliminate junk foods, sodas—colas, in particular, and sweets. It takes about five days of heebie-jeebies and then withdrawal symptoms subside—that's if you don't eat those foods, which start the craving merry-go-round all over again.

One more thing about pH

There is something that you don't eat nor drink that has great influence on the pH of your overall body. It is emotional stress: worry, fear, hate, anger, obsessions, etc. Stress does more to convert the body into an acidic state than you can ever imagine. So, if you want to be successful at changing body pH with diet, you have to consider getting your emotions under control and not worry. I know that's easier said than done. However, if you want to get well, you are going to have to work at not worrying and de-stressing your life and yourself. Please refer to Chapter 35, *Information Resources* for ideas on how to cope with stress.

Cheeseburger in Hydrochloric Acid Experiment

Brady Haran in 2010 undertook an experiment with placing a cheeseburger in pure hydrochloric acid (HCl). The experiment was performed at the University of Nottingham,

UK, and may be 'overdone' a bit, in my opinion, since no human stomach could produce as much HCl as in the beaker in the experiment. However, the video does indicate, I think, an exaggerated process of digestion for a very popular food staple. You will note that even with such an abundant concentration of HCl, some meat still does not digest.

There's also a lesson to be learned from watching the video at <ebaumsworld.com/video/watch/81084618/> about food combinations.

Food Combinations

For those with digestive problems, the art of food combining just may be what the "doctor ordered" to get digestion working efficiently. Harmonious Food Combinations are discussed in another book for which I was the writing consultant and manuscript editor, *Your Body's Diet, Where Health Begins* available on Amazon.com.

Dr Robert Jenkins, the author, states in the Summary section of Chapter Nine the following:

- *Eat fresh fruits separately or with nuts and seeds.*
- *Do not drink fruit juice with meals, period.*
- *Drink water, herbal teas, or cereal coffee sparingly—preferably not at all—when eating.*
- *Select one type of protein and one type of carbohydrate food per meal with generous servings of vegetables and raw salad (if you are able to digest raw veggies).*

- *Desserts (sweets) are eaten best once the stomach has emptied, about 1-1 ½ hours after the meal.*
- *Sweets are loners and prefer to be digested alone.*

Getting back to the cheeseburger video, the burger food combination is overloaded with protein—meat and cheese—together with a high carbohydrate white flour (starch) bun that would be in conflict with the fourth bulleted item above when considering proper food combinations. In my opinion, a slice of anemic tomato and onion with a sprig of lettuce would be nowhere near a generous serving of raw vegetables needed to balance or complement that much protein.

About High Fructose Corn Syrup [HFCS]

High fructose corn syrup is in just about every processed food product on the market. Not only does HFCS feed cancer cells, which " love and live off" sugar, HFCS is implicated in many other unhealthy conditions: diabetes, liver scarring, and obesity. This is another reason to change your eating pattern to an enzyme-rich, yeast-free diet.

Dr Jonathan V Wright, MD, in his newsletter article "HFCS linked to serious weight gain, liver scaring" reports on Princeton research done on HFCS from which the researchers concluded that HFCS is worse than fat or table sugar (sucrose). Furthermore, HFCS is *"linked to liver scarring in people with non-alcoholic fatty liver disease."*[86]

What Studies Claim About Food

Now I'm going to share with you some information about a trial study in 2005, *The Women's Healthy Eating and Living (WHEL)* study, published in *The Journal of the American Medical Association (JAMA)* wherein 3,088 women's diets were studied.

> *The women with the highest levels of carotenoids [provitamin A sources that function as antioxidants] had 43% lower chance of breast cancer recurrence or death when compared with women with the lowest levels of carotenoids in their blood.* [87]

Then another study published in *JAMA* August 15, 2007 suggests people who eat a *"Western" diet — red meat, high fat, refined grains and dessert — have a higher chance of their colon cancer returning than those who consume a "prudent" diet consisting primarily of fruits, vegetables, poultry and fish."* [88]

To which I'd like to add this last caveat: Depending upon how the poultry were raised and where the fish were caught, i.e., organically grown, free-range poultry and "wild caught," NOT farm raised fish, make all the difference in the nutritional quality of poultry and fish, including less toxic chemicals.

Reasons to Rethink a Diet High in Animal Products

Dr Michael Greger, MD, is a physician and author on nutrition, food safety, and public health issues. He also is a founding member of the American College of Lifestyle Medicine. An article he wrote and posted at *Care2* <care2.com/greenliving/stool-size-and-breast-cancer-risk.html> titled "Stool [BM] Size and Breast Cancer Risk" ought to be taken seriously by every woman regardless of whether or not she has breast cancer, in my opinion.

In that article Dr Greger points out *"Anthropologists estimate we evolved eating 100 grams of fiber a day or more!"* Remember what I said about the Paleolithic diet back in Chapter One? Greger points out that fiber helps move excess hormones and cholesterol out of the digestive tract by keeping intestinal contents flowing freely instead of getting impacted or hardening, i.e., constipation. In the article he provides an excellent analogy that I think my readers will understand immediately. Please make certain to view the 3-minute video embedded in that article titled "Relieving yourself of excess estrogen."

Another *Care2* article dramatizes the problems with meat production and animal husbandry is "Rendered Animal Wastes in Our Food Chain" at <care2.com/greenliving/rendered-animal-wastes-in-our-food-chain.html>. This, I believe, is important information that will help you understand the need for a change of diet in order to beat breast cancer. Livestock are fed rendered animal wastes, anything *"from slaughterhouse wastes, animals that died before slaughter, supermarkets and restaurants refuse, as well as waste from animal farms including manure and poultry litter."* Your body deserves better quality animal protein than that produced from such feeding practices. Grass-fed animals, in my opinion, and their food products are the only animal products that should be eaten by anyone!

There's not a vegetable that I can say I dislike, only the way it's prepared.

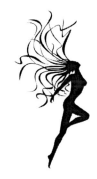

Chapter Sixteen
Nutritional Value of Unfamiliar Foods
[Those foods not eaten by most fast food addicts]

Better a meal of vegetables where there
is love than a fattened calf with hatred.

... Proverbs 15:17, *NLTB*

Vitamins and minerals are key
nutrients in making body chemistry work.

W hen I studied *natural* nutrition I learned *vitamins activate minerals.* However, the method by which food is grown and the way it is eaten can predict reliably the probable nutrient and nutritional integrity. Nutrition charts include calculated optimum nutrient content for foods. However *the importance of eating vegetables either raw or very lightly steamed* needs to be understood and practiced in order to preserve nutrients, especially raw food enzymes, so they can activate enzyme systems in your body. Overcooked, limp vegetables have little nutritional value, in my opinion, since most of the nutritional values wind up in the cooking water that you most likely pour down the kitchen sink drain.

Many readers may not be familiar with some vegetables that I talk about in this book or in the dietary section. So, here is a little *get acquainted list*, including the nutritional and life enhancing reasons for eating them.

Allium Family Vegetables
Garlic, leek, onion scallion, shallot

These high-sulfur-containing-vegetables contain several sulfur compounds, e.g., organosulfur, Allyl sulfur, and other sulfur-containing amino acids that impede cancer cell growth.

Garlic is an exceptional *natural occurring* anti-fungal that inhibits *Candida Albicans* growth in cancer patients. *Allicin* is the natural potent anti-fungal in garlic. Eating two cloves of raw garlic either on veggies or as part of the salad dressing [Recipe section] will be most beneficial as a dietary source to inhibit candida. Heat will diminish Allicin potency. If after eating raw garlic, you experience flatulence or gas, that's a rather obvious sign of some candida overgrowth in the intestinal tract. When candida gets under control you will find that raw garlic will no longer give you flatulence. Everyone must have a *correct* candida balance in our intestinal tracts for digestion, assimilation, and elimination.

Asparagus

Asparagus is considered a spring vegetable, but is available year-round because of North and South Hemispheres farming seasons and global partners.

Nutritionally, asparagus is an excellent source of Folate (B$_9$), potassium, and antioxidants, *particularly glutathione.* However, asparagus tends to give urine a strange 'sweet-like' odor, which is no cause for alarm, due to sulfur degrading compound products methyl mercaptan and asparagine.

Asparagus can be eaten lightly steamed, leftover and cold in a salad or as a side vegetable, or make cream of asparagus soup *without* dairy cream. Just place the cooled soup into a blender to cream it.

Avocado

This pear-shaped fruit, eaten as a vegetable, is an excellent source of Omega-3 and Omega-6 fatty acids. One cup of cubed avocado supplies 165 mg Omega-3 and 2534 mg Omega-6 fatty acids, which are essential in a healthful diet, besides other numerous vitamins and minerals. Avocado is a mainstay in Mexican cuisine.

Guacamole dip, made with lemon juice and raw garlic, would be an excellent source of numerous nutrients needed to get body chemistry moving. Heap guacamole on fresh vegetable slices or as an open-face sandwich spread. One medium avocado contains 4.02 grams of vegetable protein and 13.5 grams of fiber.

Burdock Root

The *root* of the burdock plant is a well known ingredient in the macrobiotic cancer management diet. Burdock root is chock full of nutrients including inulin and flavonoids, and is best known for its cleansing properties and ability to help eliminate toxins from the body—just what breast cancer patients need. It also has antifungal properties, excellent for helping contain the "yeast beast" or candida, e.g., thrush, some forms of vaginitis, something that often accompanies chemotherapy treatments due to immunosuppression, as some chemo drugs do increase the chances for infections. Also, burdock root's apparent affinity to help in the prevention of hair loss just may be helpful for those who are losing hair during chemotherapy and/or radiation treatments. Burdock root can be added to any sautéed vegetable dish, and I particularly like it in *Catherine's Special Nutrient-Rich Soup*, the recipe is in Chapter 20.

Celeriac or Celery Root

This vegetable can be an excellent substitute for potatoes. It can be cooked and mashed like potatoes or whipped into a puree. Julienned, celeriac is delicious raw on a salad or as a side raw vegetable at dinner, or as part of a snack.

Celery root is a source of magnesium, manganese, phosphorus, and potassium. Besides being a good source of dietary fiber, it contains vitamin B_6, vitamins C and K, so important in cancer management.

Cole or Brassica [Brassicaceae] Family Vegetables

These are vegetables usually from the mustard genus [*Brassicaceae*] that are high in vitamin C, and potent anticancer properties: 3,3'-diindolylmethane, sulforaphane and selenium. Cole family vegetables help repair DNA damage and retard cancer cell growth. They are an excellent source of carotenoids, especially broccoli.

Cole family vegetables include: Bok Choy (Chinese vegetable), broccoli, Broccoli Rabe, Brussels sprouts, cabbage, cauliflower, collards, kale, kohlrabi, mustard greens, radishes [Japanese *Daikon* radish, in particular, another macrobiotic staple], turnip greens, and watercress. These foods can influence cancer cell apoptosis or what's called 'cell suicide'. See Chapter One where I talk about I3C in these foods and their impact on hormone-related cancers, which breast cancer is.

Note: If you have a thyroid problem, please talk with your nutritionally oriented physician about cole family veggies in your diet. You may be advised to restrict them.

However, it is highly recommended that cancer patients eat at least a cupful of one cole family vegetable a day, and I say *twice a day*. Eat a variety over the course of a week.

Perhaps you might like to consider seriously what was said about cole/cruciferous/*Brassica* [*Brassicaceae*] family vegetables at the 2012 meeting of the American Association for Cancer Research. *HealthDay News* reported,

> *For Chinese women, consumption of cruciferous vegetables after breast cancer diagnosis is associated with improved survival in a dose-response pattern, according to a study presented at the annual meeting of the American Association for Cancer Research, held from March 31 to April 4* [2012] *in Chicago. …*

"Commonly consumed cruciferous vegetables in China include turnips, Chinese cabbage/bok choy, and greens, while broccoli and brussels sprouts are the more-consumed cruciferous vegetables in the United States and other Western countries," Necuhuta said in a statement. "Second, the amount of intake among Chinese women is much higher than that of U.S. women. The level of bioactive compounds such as isothiocyanates and indoles, proposed to play a role in the anticancer effects of cruciferous vegetables, depend on both the amount and type of cruciferous vegetables consumed." [89a]

Kale [Two Varieties: green and red]

Kale is a leafy vegetable that can be eaten raw in salad or *lightly steamed.* It's a good source of fiber, plus calcium, copper, iron, magnesium, manganese, phosphorus, and potassium.

Kale is a rich source of the following vitamins: A, Thiamin (B_1), Riboflavin (B_2), Pyridoxine (B_6), Folate (B_9), and vitamin K. Note: *Folic acid is the synthetic form of Folate B_9.*

One cup of Kale provides the Daily Value (DV) for the following minerals:

26% DV manganese, 10% DV copper, 9% calcium and potassium each, 6% iron and magnesium each, 4% phosphorus, 2% zinc, 1% selenium and sodium each.

Pumpkin

Most folks are familiar with pumpkin pie, the traditional Thanksgiving dinner dessert. However, it's jam-packed with white sugar in most cases, which is not conducive to reducing cancer-producing cells in the body, since cancer cells just 'love' sugar and any edibles and starches that convert into sugar during the digestive processes.

Pumpkins are members of *cururbitaceae* family, similar to cantaloupes, cucumbers, and other squashes, e.g., cocozelle, crooknecks, zucchini. Some squashes are now GMO. Be careful to eat organically grown zucchini and yellow squash, as squashes have been genetically modified.

Raw pumpkin is rich in antioxidants, e.g., alpha carotene and other carotenoids, and contains Omega-3 fatty acids (in the form of alpha-linolenic acid [ALA]) and Omega 6-fatty acids; abounds in potassium, plus numerous minerals; complex B vitamins, and virtually sodium free in *its natural state.* That's why it's better *to steam* fresh pumpkin and eat it as a steamed vegetable.

After cleaning a pumpkin, consider using the seeds. Wash, pat dry, and place them on a baking pan in a warm oven (200°F) for about 10 minutes; remove and let cool. Store in a glass jar in the refrigerator and eat as a snack, or as a crunchy topping on a green salad. Those wonderful tasting seeds provide zinc, selenium, and the amino acid L-tryptophan.

Canned pumpkin, however, is reduced in nutrient content due to processing techniques. However, it still is a valued food item that can be used to make pumpkin pudding as a dessert or snack food. See my recipe for *Pumpkin Custard Pudding* in the Recipe section in Chapter 20.

This information about canned pumpkin ought to be a valuable indicator of the importance of fresh, raw, and lightly steamed vegetables in any cancer management diet.

Root Vegetables

Root vegetables are those that grow underground as bulbs, corms, rhizomes, or tubers.

Potatoes probably are the most familiar root vegetable. If you eat potatoes daily or other root vegetables in great quantity, you must re-evaluate that habit and change to eating more leafy green and low *Glycemic Index* veggies so as to eliminate starches and naturally occurring sugars that convert into high sugar values in the body, which excites candida growth and 'fertilizes' cancer cells.

According to the *Glycemic Index* (GI), a listing of 70 and above is HIGH; 56-69 is medium; and 55 and under is low. French fries have a GI index of 75; a baked potato comes in at 85; and instant mashed potatoes, 86.

However, a yam or sweet potato has a lower GI when boiled as opposed to a much higher GI when baked. The method of cooking changes how naturally occurring sugars in vegetables are gelatinized and/or caramelized during cooking. That's something you will want to keep in mind with regard to food preparation and cooking.

Sea Vegetables - Seaweed

Kombu (*Laminaria japonica*), in particular, is very important in the macrobiotic dietary approach to managing cancers. This dried sea vegetable contains fiber, vitamins A and B_1; the minerals calcium, iron, magnesium, phosphorus, potassium; glutamic acid, an amino acid that enhances taste; and the trace element, iodine.

Some additional beneficial nutrients in sea vegetables include: alginate compounds, antioxidants, Omega-3 and Omega-6 fatty acids, flavonoids, *Fucoidan, Laminarin,* plant sterols, polyphenols, and trace minerals. Seaweed probably is the most important food source for balanced *trace* minerals.

Other dried, edible seaweeds include *Arame, Hijiki, Nori,* and *Wakame.*

May I share with you a famous story about the use of seaweed in Japan after the 1945 atomic bombings?

> *In 1945, at the time of the atomic bombing of Japan, Dr. Tatsuichiro Akizuki was Director of the Department of Internal Medicine at St. Francis's Hospital in Nagasaki. Most patients in the hospital, which was located one mile from the center of the blast, survived the initial effects of the bomb – but came down with symptoms of radiation sickness from the fallout.*
>
> *The doctor fed his staff and patients a strict diet consisting of: brown rice, miso and tamari soy soup, wakame, kombu and other seaweed, Hokkaido pumpkin, and sea salt. He prohibited the consumption of sugar and sweets to help prevent radiation sickness from pre-existing exposure.*
>
> *Dr. Akizuki saved everyone in his hospital, while many others in the area died from radiation sickness.* [89]

If you have had radiation treatments, perhaps *Kombu* and *Wakame* should be included in your diet. Just two one-inch sections of *Kombu* a day are sufficient. Eat it as you would popcorn. You also can use it to flavor soups and other recipes.

For more information about seaweed, please see Chapter 27, *Sea Vegetables & Fucoidan.*

Walnuts [English *not* Black]

These *raw* nuts make excellent snacking foods instead of junk foods or high carbohydrate edibles you may have been used to eating. According to research done at Marshall University, a daily dose of walnuts in mice that equaled 2 ounces a day in humans was correlated with reducing breast cancer tumor growth in mice. [90]

Walnuts are a high source of Omega 3-fatty acids. Would you believe that just one-quarter (¼) cup of walnuts provides close to 91 percent of the recommended daily value for Omega-3s?

Raw walnuts are an exceptionally good source of the B complex vitamins plus vitamin E, an antioxidant. I suggest keeping *organic* walnuts in a glass jar in the refrigerator. You can add them to salads for crunch and taste and, as I like, to hot oatmeal cereal with some cinnamon and organic coconut milk for a yummy breakfast that has a staying power of about six hours, at least for me.

Also, if after eating a meal you don't feel satiated—or satisfied—eat a small handful of English walnuts as dessert and see how quickly you feel full.

Dr Michael Greger, MD, a founding member of the American College of Lifestyle Medicine, has a rather interesting

YouTube video, *#1 AntiCancer Vegetables,* at <youtube.com/ watch?feature=player_embedded&v=8tAAehC4BYs#1>.

As you view it, please keep in mind what I've said about vegetables in this chapter.

Oh, how interesting to find something new in life.

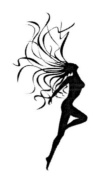

Chapter Seventeen
Particleboard-like Food

Don't eat anything your great-great grandmother wouldn't recognize as food. There are a great many food-like items in the supermarket your ancestors wouldn't recognize as food (Go-Gurt? Breakfast-cereal bars? Nondairy creamer?); stay away from these.

... Michael Pollan (1955—)
Author, *The Omnivore's Dilemma*

What is particleboard-like food? you probably are asking.

*I*t's my definition of most processed food. If you are familiar with particleboard, you know that it

> *is an engineered wood product manufactured from wood particles, such as wood chips, sawmill shavings, or even saw dust, and a synthetic resin or other suitable binder, which is pressed and extruded. Particleboard is a composite material.* [91]

That description not only defines particleboard but, in my opinion, also is a perfect descriptive parallel for today's modern processed foods sold in supermarkets, grocery, and convenience stores, I think. Often such edibles are referred to as convenience foods, junk foods, and snacks, which many people eat as their primary diet.

The food processing industry has taken food to the next level of composite materials and degeneration, in my opinion, when they remove vital nutrients during milling and/or processing, and then adds synthetic ones, as is done with synthetic B vitamin enrichment in milled white flours—a high glycemic value starch. White bread has a Glycemic Index value of 70. Wheat's nutritious food components—wheat germ and bran—are extracted and often sold as separate health or enrichment products, or as farm animal feed enhancements. To learn more about the *Glycemic Index,* may I suggest your checking out the Harvard School of Public Health's informative website at <hsph.Harvard.edu/nutritionsource/what-should-you-eat/carbohydratres/>.

Furthermore, food processors love to add all sorts of synthetic ingredients, artificial flavors, colors, monosodium glutamate—even if it's not listed on the label, it is there in what I call "MSG clones"—and a host of synthetic chemically-produced ingredients your grandma wouldn't recognize. Most ingredients, by law, must be and are listed within the ingredient label. Unfortunately, many times some things 'slip through' as the article "Chocolate Drink Recalled: Undeclared Wheat" verifies and, luckily, there was a product recall listed. [92] One of the things slipping through because of the U.S. FDA directive is GMO ingredients; they are not listed on labels.

An ingredient label usually is your first clue to particleboard-like food. However, product advertising and package displays tout how nutritious the product is *supposed* to be. How can that be when, in most instances, there is not enough real food content in the product to provide real food nutritional values? An excellent example comes from the Health Ranger, Mike Adams, wherein he critiques blueberries, which aren't real blueberries but composites made of sugars, hydrogenated vegetable oils, artificial flavors and colors, etc. I encourage you to visit <natural.news.tv/v.asp?v=7EC06D27B1A945BE8 5E7DA8483025962> for an extraordinary tutorial. Here's an excerpt from that video.

> *Pictures of blueberries are prominently displayed on the front of many food packages. Here they are on boxes of muffins, cereals and breads. But turn the packages around, and suddenly the blueberries disappear. They're gone, replaced in the ingredients list with sugars, oils and artificial colors derived from petrochemicals.*
>
> *This bag of blueberry bagels sold at Target stores is made with blueberry bits. And while actual blueberries are found further down the ingredients list, the blueberry bits themselves don't even contain bits of blueberries. They're made entirely from sugar, corn cereal, modified food starch, partially hydrogenated vegetable oil, artificial flavor, cellulose gum, salt and artificial colors like Blue #2, Red #40, Green #3 and Blue #1.*

*What's missing from that list? Well, blueberries.
Where did the blueberries go? …*

The above is only one example, probably a classic at that. How about going into your kitchen or pantry and start reading labels on processed food products and see what you find. How much real food really is in a product? With very little, if any at all enzymes, vitamins—other than synthetic ones— minerals, fiber, and other nutrients that are processed out, and chemical ingredients substituted or added, what is there that your body's cells can use for nutrition besides chemicals, sugar, and starchy carbohydrates? Therein lies the problem with particleboard-like food—the composite materials don't contribute nutrients or nutritional value, but starve cells that must, in turn, go scrounging for food to live, thrive, and multiply. When no nutrients are found, unfortunately they mutate in order to 'survive and thrive' as cancer cells.

When cells don't find the nutrients they need, they start reprogramming themselves into other ways to 'do business' in the body, which usually ends in abnormal cell production, e.g., cancerous cells and/or tumors. A similar scenario takes place when you are exposed to chemicals that damage DNA, and that's almost every synthetically-produced petrochemical used in all phases of commerce from clothing to mattresses to furniture to flooring to cabinetry to cosmetics—you name it, and food! Lastly, improper acid/alkaline [pH] balance also encourages cancerous cell growth. Particleboard-like foods definitely convert into an acid ash within the body.

To understand the physiology of cancer to a certain degree, one must realize that cancer starts as a result of cells either being damaged beyond repair, usually at DNA telomeres, or by cells literally starving and unable to carry on healthy lifestyles for lack of nutrition and then reprogramming themselves to 'alternative life cycles' by living off organisms like yeast, fungus, and other microorganisms that evolve in an acidic pH body chemistry from dietary trash circulating and being used as 'nutrition'. To understand what I just said, here's a quick overview of how nutrition is delivered to cells.

> *Nutrients absorbed through the intestinal membranes are delivered in the blood circulation and transported to all tissues and organs, where they are absorbed by the cells.* [93] [Cells also absorb chemicals and toxins from particleboard-like food since most human livers are compromised now because of the daily onslaught of toxins.]

For readers who are not located near organically grown food sources and are wondering how to purchase organic food, you may want to know about a company that is dedicated not only to growing organic foods but also to an organic lifestyle. I have no financial interests in the company nor do they know that I'm recommending them in my book. However, I do feel that **Beyond Organics** just may be what you are looking for. You may find them online at <beyondorganicinsider.com/becomeaninsider.aspx?enroller=47912>.

Before I leave the concept of particleboard-like food, I'd like to point out that the holistic health community has been discussing, growing, selling, and eating real foods for a healthful lifestyle ever since I can remember. Weren't they/we the original "health nuts"? Back in the 1980s I recall a medical doctor telling me, *"If there was anything to nutrition, don't you think we'd know about it."* So what does that remark say about their being up to date and knowledge about issues? How much nutrition education did they get in med school then? Maybe an hour! Not much has changed. Recently I heard about one of the medical associations complaining about MDs having to receive 8 Continuing Ed credits in nutrition.

But the food ladies in hospitals—registered dietitians, at that time were 'up in arms' about getting licensed to be the only professionals to dispense nutrition information. I remember testifying before several state legislature committee hearings on such licensure—often with the late Dr Robert S Mendelsohn, MD (1926-1988)—that RDs should NOT have monopolistic licensure, which violated free speech rights, and because what RDs did, in essence, was promote the food processing industry's spin on food, which was abysmal factual information about nutrition then and some still is, in my opinion. White bread was really good for you. Really?

Furthermore, I had fun introducing into the record, the RD exam cram book and some of the questions that were asked on exams about supposed nutrition, e.g., how to prepare gelatin for 500 people. First of all, gelatin is not one of the 'foods' I nor any *natural* nutritionist would recommend for a sick person because it is ground up offal, bones, and often slaughterhouse floor sweepings—yuck, plus sugar and food coloring.

But as holistic life styles became more prominent and grocery store chains like Fresh Fields, Whole Foods, and Trader Joe came along, consumers began to appreciate wholesome and organically grown foods. Registered dietitians reluctantly began to embrace our way of thinking about nutrients in food—but as I believe—are still in the 'back pocket' of the big food processing industry, which supports many of their projects, as I had heard confirmed during testimonies made by registered dieticians in the 1980s at licensing hearings. I don't think much has changed about food processing industry support for RDs. However, I must congratulate RDs on their apparent reading of our natural nutrition literature and making some concessions.

Today, as I listen to radio advertisements hawking medical proficiencies, I hear medical spin masters promoting such advances as hospitals and medical practices that promote "*culinary medicine*." Wow! Those are impressive words with a possible correct conceptualization, I'd say. However, I don't think it amounts to much nutritionally. Why? Because when it comes to providing food and nutrition guidance, the allopathic paradigm still relies upon the food processing and industrial kitchen industries, especially in the promotion of *chemically processed* and *genetically modified foods*. What does that tell you about culinary medicine? In my opinion, you—and they— will know when real culinary medicine happens, as inpatient hospital meals and food service will be totally different from the 'fast food' concept of fried and steam table edibles, plus fast food restaurants no longer will set up business within hospital cafeterias.

If only we knew how enzyme-packed fresh raw food can be, we then would know the road to health and wellness.

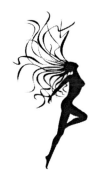

Chapter Eighteen

A Nutritional Case AGAINST Chocolate

Researchers have discovered that chocolate produces some of the same reactions in the brain as marijuana. The researchers also discovered other similarities between the two but can't remember what they are.

…Matt Lauer (1957—)
TV Personality

Contrary to claims that chocolate is an excellent source of phytochemicals and antioxidants, there is a downside to cocoa and chocolate that needs to be considered when eating to manage breast cancer, or any cancer, I think.

Here is some information you may not know about chocolate that can make a difference in your approach to the management of any disease, but breast cancer in particular—or any cancer. Since most chocolate contains sugar or a synthetic sugar substitute or derivative, which excites yeast production and *candida* in the body, chocolate definitely should be avoided, I say.

Chocolate is the product of a fermentation process to cocoa beans, which are roasted and become 'sweeter' instead of having their original bitter taste. This is done by placing cocoa beans between layers of banana leaves for seven or more days, depending upon how much chocolate aroma is produced. Then the fermented *cacao beans are sometimes treated by alkali in a process called "Dutching". This process removes some of the acidity of the beans and gives a more smooth flavor and a darker color of the cocoa.* [94]

The Cocoa Bean is the source of Chocolate, which can be:

- Habit forming; craving it may mean a chromium and magnesium deficiency and an indicator of blood sugar metabolism problems
- A mild stimulant
- A mood elevator for hyperactivity and nervousness
- A high allergy food
- A trigger source for other allergic reactions, e.g., migraine headaches, hives
- **Note:** *there's some indication theobromine in chocolate can help relieve asthma attacks though.*
- A source of theobromine, which is similar to caffeine (an alkaloid; xantheose) and the reason dogs and other pets can die from eating chocolate
- Cocoa beans naturally contain between 300-1200 mg *per ounce of theobromine* depending upon bean quality

- A possible risk/connection to prostate cancer in older men from theobromines
- A source of phenethylamine, which can produce psychological effects in humans
- A source of toxic pesticide residues because of agricultural practices used, e.g.,
  - ○ **Methyl Bromide** — *prostate cancer, kidney and liver effects, neurological effects*
  - ○ **Pyrethrins** — *carcinogenicity, reproductive and developmental toxicity, neurotoxicity*
  - ○ **Hydrogen Cyanide** — *acute toxicity, thyroid effects, nerve degeneration*
  - ○ **Naled** — *central nervous system disruption; headaches, nausea and diarrhea*
  - ○ **Glyphosate** — *effects on digestive system tissue, genetic damage, effects on reproduction, carcinogenicity* [Glyphosate is used in/on GMO crops]

Lindane—a pesticide best known for use as a treatment for head lice—is banned in the US for use on food crops but has been found to be a contaminant in some European chocolate. [95]

Cadmium and lead have been found at significant levels in 68% of chocolate products tested by the American Environmental Safety Institute. Cadmium is a well-known carcinogen. Lead is unsafe at any level, and children are particularly affected by it. [96]

Note: The EPA allows certain levels of pesticides in cocoa powder/chocolate.[96]

Sulfuryl fluoride, an anti-termite insecticide, has been an approved cacao fumigant that EPA is working to phase out of cocoa-chocolate and other foods, e.g., *non-organic* walnuts. Are you beginning to realize the importance of organically grown food?

As for organically grown cocoa and chocolate, even though not subject to toxic growing methods, it should be avoided until the remission stage of breast or any cancer is accomplished, and then only *minimal* consumption, in my opinion.

All of the evil that people have thrust upon chocolate is really more deserved by milk chocolate, which is essentially contaminated. The closer you get to a pure chocolate liquor (the chocolate essence ground from roasted cacao beans) the purer it is, the more satisfying it is, the safer it is, and the healthier it is.
...Arnold Ismach, "The Darker Side of Chocolate"

To which I ask, "Isn't there sugar in everything chocolate?"

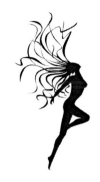

Chapter Nineteen
Foods High in Sulfur

Special Note Regarding Food Allergies

*I*t is important *NOT* to eat any foods to which you have food allergies, as doing that places strain on the immune system which, of course, you want to avoid since you are trying to build up the immune system as quickly as possible.

Daily Vegetables
[Eat at least *7 vegetables—preferably more*—a day from this selection]

Allium family members:
    Chives, garlic*, leeks, onions*, shallots, scallions
Asparagus (glutathione)
Avocado
Brassica or Cole-family vegetables
    Bok Choy, broccoli, Brussels sprouts, cabbage, cauli-flower, watercress

Collard greens

Kale

Legumes

    Beans, lentils (methionine), peas

Methionine amino acid in

    Grains: Corn, oats; *Nuts:* Almonds, walnuts; *Seeds:*
Sesame seeds

Mustard greens

Parsley

Radishes [long white Daikon radish, in particular]

Sauerkraut

Swiss Chard

Tomatoes

Yams [only once a week, boiled not baked because of sugars
in yams]

    * Studies indicate that phytochemicals (plant chemicals)
in garlic and onions have been shown to increase T-cell
activity and, interestingly, aged garlic seems to work even
better.

    Only animal protein I suggest until body is stabilized:
organic eggs

    When FRUIT Is Introduced *[usually after 3 months on the
diet]* I waited 6 months.

    Apples, organic preferred

Berries: Blueberries, Blackberries, Raspberries, and
Strawberries [organic preferably]

    Melons very infrequently

    Pears [organic preferably]

When Meat & Fish Are Introduced

Depending upon how advanced the cancer is, meat and fish may not be on your menu for a while, I suggest, since a strict vegetarian diet seems to work most effectively to eradicate cancer cells and/or retard their growth.

Red meats: grass fed, organically grown once a week, if at all

Chicken: *ONLY organically grown* strictly twice a week, if at all

Numerous holistic cancer treatment researchers and physicians report that meat seems to re-activate tumor growth. Dr Max Gerson found that meat and fats, in particular, did just that, so that's why the Gerson protocol is strictly vegetarian.

White flesh fishes—no tuna, swordfish, mackerel [all high in mercury], NO shellfish

Raw Foods

Femtalk USA – Cancer Section, "Foods That Fight Cancer" online at <femtalkusa.com/cancer7.htm> states that a 70 percent raw food (uncooked) diet is recommended. Others think a 50 percent raw food diet is sufficient. Personally, I believe the diet should be as much raw food as you can eat, which ought to be closer to 70 percent. Juicing fresh green vegetables counts as raw food.

Also, I'd like to suggest getting familiar with T cell information online at *MedicineNet* at <medterms.com/script/main/art.asp?articlekey=11300>. I think it will help you understand and appreciate what comes into play with regard to the immune system.

Why Such A Fixation on Sulfur Foods?

Foods containing generous amounts of sulfur have a detoxi-fying effect on the body, fortify the immune system, counter-act aging, and help relieve the effects of some chronic diseases like arthritis. Most of those aspects certainly come into play when dealing with breast cancer.

Sulfur is an essential mineral component in protein foods—especially organically grown, pasture-raised hen eggs, plus vitamin B$_1$ (Thiamine), biotin, and the amino acids methionine, cysteine, taurine, and glutathione. Depending upon freshness, the pH of an egg white is 9 [alkaline] while the yolk is 6.5, slightly acid. Remember pH 7 is neutral. Even though the classification for eggs is acid, based upon individual pH for the white and the yolk, when averaged out since most eggs are eaten with both the white and yolk, it sug-gests that an organically grown egg may be more alkaline in ash, in my opinion.

Scientifically speaking, most animal proteins are consid-ered acid. Another issue to keep in mind about non-organ-ically-raised hens and their eggs is that the living conditions under which they are housed lead to their bodies creating a lot of stress hormones that, in turn, impact the nutritional and pH value—I'd venture to say really acid—of their eggs. But, again, that's my opinion.

The best cooking method for high-sulfur-containing veg-etables is blanching, steaming in a steamer basket, or *low heat* cooking for longer periods of time, e.g., lentils and beans.

Never discard any high-sulfur vegetable cooking water; drink it like an herbal tea. Add a tad of sea salt to make it more like a vegetable broth.

Don't cook the enzymes out of vegetables; they should have crunch, which means nutrients are still in them and enzymes are active as you eat them.

Note: If there is any cooking liquid left over in the steamer pot, let it cool, add a tad of sea salt and drink all those valuable nutrients that you would have washed down the drain.

Eat to live—don't live to eat.

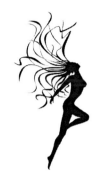

Chapter Twenty
Sample Menu Planning Ideas With Recipes

Leave your drugs in the chemist's pot if you can heal the patient with food.

… Hippocrates (c.460BCE—370BCE)
The Father of Modern Medicine

A Note Regarding Food Allergies

*I*t is most important NOT to eat foods to which you have known food allergies, as doing that places strain on the immune system which, of course, you want to avoid since you are eating and working to build up the immune system.

The *Recipe* section follows the sample menus below. You will find—and hopefully enjoy—my special recipes for yeast- and vinegar-free, gourmet-tasty, food preparation.

As a retired *natural* nutritionist who treasures the value of real food nutrients, I'd like to share with you some meal plans I designed and ate during my holistic breast cancer treatment. I think they may give you some idea of how easy and tasty a holistic breast cancer treatment diet really can be. Also, so easy to prepare.

Breakfast

#1B Fruit [choose only one from this selection]
- Lightly stewed or raw organic apple [cut into 8ths] with organic walnuts
- Baked organic apple stuffed with organic walnuts and cinnamon with side dressing of organic light coconut milk or rice milk or almond milk [optional]
- Raw organic apple slices spread with organic almond butter
- *Note:* No fruit other than apple for the first six months on the program, I suggest. That's what I did. After that I introduced organic strawberries, blackberries, and champagne mangoes (small yellow mangoes).

#2B Cereal
Cooked—not instant—organic oatmeal with ¼ cup organic walnut pieces, cinnamon, and organic light coconut milk [You could substitute almond, oat, or rice milk; *no soy* as most soy is GMO. Furthermore, soy is a high allergy food and can produce negative effects on the thyroid for some people.]

#3B
Organic egg soft cooked [4 minutes means cooked white with a runny yolk]

Sourdough/yeast-free *whole grain bread* with a tad of organic *no sugar* fruit spread (not compatible for food combining) or organic almond butter spread, **OR**

homemade *organic cornbread* with organic almond butter instead of dairy butter

#4B

Bowl of *Catherine's Special Nutrient-Rich Soup* with one slice of sourdough/yeast-free organic *whole grain bread* spread with organic almond butter, OR homemade *organic cornbread*

#5B

Any leftovers from dinner with cornbread and almond butter

Lunch

#1L

Mug of *Cream of Asparagus, Gazpacho* Soup, or *Catherine's Special Nutrient-Rich Soup*

Only one rice cake *OR one* slice of yeast-free whole grain bread to make an open face sandwich heaped with a generous amount of

Eggplant Pâté topped with organic tomato slices and organic Arugula sprouts

Herbamare seasoning and Cayenne pepper to taste

Hijiki Seaweed Salad or *Cucumber Salad*

6 to 8 oz fresh pressed green juice made from organ-ically grown

1 medium cucumber

4 green kale leaves

5 Romaine lettuce leaves

1 green zucchini

¼ bunch parsley

1 lime

For some zip, you can add a ½ inch piece of fresh ginger root.

1 Tablespoon cold pressed organic high lignan flaxseed oil

For readers who are not familiar with juicing, you may want to check out "Favorite Green Juice Recipes" online at <prolifi-cliving.com/blog/2009/04/13/favorite-green-juice-recipes/>. To juice vegetables, you will need to purchase a masticating juicer. Have fun juicing.

#2L

Mug of *Cream of Asparagus, Gazpacho* Soup, or *Catherine's Special Nutrient-Rich Soup*

Only one rice cake *OR one* slice of yeast-free whole grain bread to make an open face sandwich heaped with one sliced hard cooked organic egg, tomato slices and Arugula sprouts

A side serving of raw Daikon radish

Herbamare seasoning and Cayenne pepper to taste

Hijiki Seaweed Salad or *Cucumber Salad*

6 to 8 oz any freshly pressed green juice

1 Tablespoon cold pressed organic high lignan flaxseed oil

#3L
Hummus Wrap

Organic *non-GMO* corn tortilla spread with organic *Hummus* topped with organic avocado, sliced organic Heirloom tomato, and Arugula sprouts

Cup of *Catherine's Special Nutrient-Rich Soup*

Any leftover steamed vegetables can be eaten cold: asparagus, broccoli, cauliflower, green beans, kale

1 Tablespoon cold pressed organic high lignan flaxseed oil

#4L
Veggie Wrap

Organic *non-GMO* corn tortilla stuffed with organic avocado, organic tomato slices, Arugula (my favorite) or other sprouts, 2 or 3 Heirloom lettuce leaves, a sprinkling of lime juice, Herbamare OR sea salt, and Cayenne pepper.

Cup of *Cream of Asparagus, Gazpacho* Soup, or *Catherine's Special Nutrient-Rich Soup*

Handful of organic walnuts

1 Tablespoon cold pressed organic high lignan flaxseed oil

#5L
Stuffed Taco Shells

2 Organic *non-GMO* corn taco shells heated in 250°F toaster oven for 3 minutes to freshen

Stuff each taco shell with 2 heaping Tablespoons of:

. *Guacamole* **OR**
. Eggplant dip / *Baba Ganoush* **OR**
. *Hummus*
   Add:
. *Chopped* organic onions, organic tomato cubes, organic lettuce, organic avocado, and organic cucumber
6 to 8 oz fresh pressed green juice
1 Tablespoon cold pressed organic high lignan flaxseed oil

#6L

Vegetable Stuffed Tortillas
2 Organic *non-GMO* corn tortillas heated in a 250°F oven for 3 minutes to freshen
Stuff with
. Sliced organic avocado (1/2 avocado in each tortilla)
. Chopped organic sweet onion
. Organic tomato slices
. Organic Heirloom lettuce shredded
. Thin sweet red pepper slices
. Grated green zucchini
6 to 8 oz fresh pressed green juice
1 Tablespoon cold pressed organic high lignan flaxseed oil

#7L

Leftover Stir-Fry Open face Sandwich
Re-heat *stir-fry* [Recipe section]. Spoon over yeast-free whole grain slice of bread to make an open face sandwich. Top

with sliced organic tomato and fresh sprouts. I particularly like Arugula sprouts.

Serve with half a ripe organic avocado and some *Harvard red beet salad* [Recipe section]

1 Tablespoon cold pressed organic high lignan flaxseed oil

#8L

Crudités Platter

Wash and cut into slices, raw organic vegetables:

¼ red or yellow sweet pepper

2 radishes or part of a Daikon radish

1 rib of celery

1 small *thin* carrot

4 cherry tomatoes cut in half

Arrange veggie slices on a dinner plate with a ramekin of *Baba Ganoush* [Recipe section] OR *Hummus* [Recipe section]. Eat as vegetable dip.

Six *yeast-free* crackers, e.g., *Mary's Gone Crackers* Organic Wheat-Free Gluten-Free Caraway Crispy Crackers. Make certain any crackers are yeast-free and organic.

1 Tablespoon cold pressed organic high lignan flaxseed oil

#9L

The Quintessential Wrap Sandwich

Organic *non-GMO* corn tortilla spread with

a heaping tablespoon of *Baba Ganoush*, then layered with sliced organic avocado

sliced organic tomato (Heirlooms are delish!)

topped with sautéed red peppers and onions leftovers [Recipe section]

Arugula sprouts

1 Romaine lettuce leaf

Roll up the wrap and enjoy. The yum factor is truly delicious. Make two because only one will haunt you.

1 Tablespoon cold pressed organic high lignan flaxseed oil

Dinner

#1D

Large bowl of *Catherine's Special Nutrient-Rich Soup*

Sourdough organic whole grain bread 1 slice

Steamed organic asparagus

Sliced organic tomatoes with garlic/lemon/parsley dressing

Daikon radish slices

Freshly pressed juice [optional]

2 one-inch pieces *Kombu* seaweed

1 Tablespoon cold pressed organic high lignan flaxseed oil

#2D

Hijiki Seaweed salad [Recipe section]

Small organic Red Bliss potato baked served either dry or with *Eggplant dip/ Pâté* topping

Small organic Heirloom tomato sliced and sprinkled with *Herbamare* topped with chopped organic parsley, lime juice, and organic olive oil

Steamed green beans

Teacup of *Gazpacho* cold soup

2 one-inch pieces *Kombu* seaweed

1 Tablespoon cold pressed organic high lignan flaxseed oil

#3D

Egg Frittata (Potato-onion or Zucchini-onion) [Recipe section]

Vegetables, lightly steamed/blanched: Asparagus, Brussels sprouts, broccoli, cauliflower, collards, kale, green beans Italiano [at least 3 veggies]

Tomatoes sliced topped with garlic/lemon/parsley dressing

2 one-inch pieces *Kombu* seaweed

1 Tablespoon cold pressed organic high lignan flaxseed oil

#4D

Hard cooked organic egg sliced

Vegetables as at #3D above served with side of *Eggplant dip*

Cucumber Salad [Recipe section]

2 one-inch pieces *Kombu* seaweed

1 Tablespoon cold pressed organic high lignan flaxseed oil

#5D

Vegetable Stir-Fry [Recipe section]

One *medium to small* size baked organic potato (Red Bliss is very tasty)

Green salad with lemon or limejuice and organic olive oil drizzle

2 one-inch pieces *Kombu* seaweed

1 Tablespoon cold pressed organic high lignan flaxseed oil

#6D

2 *Quinoa Stuffed Zucchini Boats* (1 entire zucchini) [Recipe section]

Perfect Green Salad [Recipe section] with organic cherry tomatoes, limejuice, and organic olive oil

Handful of organic English walnuts

2 one-inch pieces *Kombu* seaweed

1 Tablespoon cold pressed organic high lignan flaxseed oil

#7D

Garbanzo Bean Stew [Recipe section]

Perfect Green Salad with limejuice

Asparagus lightly steamed

2 one-inch pieces *Kombu* seaweed

1 Tablespoon cold pressed organic high lignan flaxseed oil

Desserts

- Organic Gunpowder green tea
- Organic Red Clover tea
- *Pau D'Arco* tea
- Home made *organic corn bread* [Recipe section] with *no sugar* fruit preserves
- *Pumpkin Custard Pudding* [Recipe section]

Two Hours Later Dessert: Lightly stewed organic apples topped with organic walnuts

Snacks

- Organic rice cake (only 1) spread with *Hummus* or Eggplant Dip (*Baba Ganoush*) topped with tomato slices and sprouts, or cherry tomatoes on the side
- Raw vegetables, e.g., sliced cucumber, sliced Daikon radish, sweet red pepper slices, cherry tomatoes, scallions, with *Hummus* or *Eggplant Dip*
- Freshly pressed green vegetable juice
- Organic rice cake (only 1) spread with organic almond butter
- Cup of *Catherine's Special Nutrient-Rich Soup*
- Cup of *Gazpacho*
- *Pumpkin Custard Pudding* ramekin topped with organic walnut pieces
- Organic English walnuts
- Organic Brazil nuts [source of bioavailable selenium]
- Organic raw or baked apple with organic walnuts

Recipes

A Word About Food Preparation and Cooking

Safety

It is important to remember that cleanliness is paramount in preparing food. It's a safe habit to wash hands with soap and warm/hot water as often as possible during any food preparing process, especially after you have changed from preparing one food to another, e.g., chicken then vegetables, eggs then bread, fruit then veggies, etc.

In order to retain nutrients, vegetables should be very crunchy and not cooked long or overcooked, i.e., don't cook the life and nutrition out of them. Don't caramelize vegetables. Don't blacken foods using any type of fat, e.g., butter or oil. Fats when burned produce free radicals, which are cancer-causing agents.

Also, please remember if something doesn't look, smell, or feel right—when in doubt—throw it out!

Pots 'n Pans

The pots and pans in which you make soup, steam vegetables, or bake in an oven definitely can impact food's toxic quality insofar as toxins from cooking vessels can migrate from pots or pans into the food due to a chemical reaction with heat, water, and the pH of food within the cooking vessel.

A classic example to visually understand that is to cook tomatoes in an aluminum pot. First, if you do this experiment, *please don't eat the tomatoes,* as they will contain aluminum, which is a neurotoxin. However, you will see that the aluminum pot where the tomatoes cooked is a totally different and vibrant aluminum color, whereas the pot above the tomato line is a much darker color, which means some aluminum migrated from the pot into the tomatoes.

The safest cooking pots, pans, and oven-safe roasting pans, I think, are made of stove-top and oven-proof glass, real porcelain-covered ironware (e.g., LeCreuset French cookware is a safe brand that I've used since shortly after getting married), and good quality stainless steel, which is a combination of iron, chromium, nickel, sometimes manganese or molybdenum—depending upon type and grade of stainless steel manufactured and cooking use—that theoretically could leach out metals if not manufactured correctly. Stainless steel food utensils are graded several ways: 18/8, 18/10, and the 300 series. The 18/10 or 304 grades usually are the safest in pots and pans.

By no means do I recommend plastic coated or plastic enamel-like cookware even though they may have pretty designs on them; non-stick cookware; aluminum pots and/or pans; cardboard or paperboard containers; or silicone because of the possibility of dye colors migrating out during high heat interactions. To understand the problems with non-stick cookware, please study the online information "Skip the non-stick to avoid the dangers of Teflon" at <ewg.org/healthyhometips/dangersofteflon>.

Microwave Cooking

Here's where I probably am going to lose you. However, I must be true not only to myself but you, if conquering cancer is the goal. First and foremost, I must confess I never bought into microwave cooking from day one. I never had a microwave unit in any kitchen in a house that my late husband and I owned, nor in my present townhouse.

Besides the documented scientific studies of harm microwaves do to cooks who use them, e.g., eye problems, microwaves are a form of radiation—see the chart in Chapter 9, *Radiation: What Is It*. Microwave low frequency radiation has to affect whatever is exposed to it, regardless of what proponents say. Recall all the controversy over the years about cell phone radiation. Does it or does it not produce brain tumors? That depends upon whatever you want to believe. For me, I must confess from all my studies and research I've come to the conclusion, "better be safe than sorry."

One thing I know for certain is what happens to me when I eat microwave-cooked food: I get constipated for days—something I never experience otherwise or have during my life. Usually that happened when I would eat out either at friends' houses or in a restaurant, which was not often, except during travel time. That tells me that my body cannot handle microwaved food as normal food, and my digestive processes are screwed up because of some apparent biochemical foul-up. I listen to my body when it talks to me and try to figure out what's going on.

Having made my confession about microwave cooking, that's all I will say. However, there have been some experiments done over the years with plants fed microwaved water that have been pooh-poohed as unscientific. Well, all I can say is do your own experiment and see what happens in your kitchen. If you would like to read an online article about such an experiment, you may find it at <naturalnews.com/031929_ microwaved_water_plants.html>.

Plastic

In my opinion, plastic does not belong near food or in the kitchen as food containers. It's made with many toxic chemicals that can and do migrate because of heat temperature and pH values in food. For food storage, use washed and dried glass jars with screw top or pop top lids to store food in cabinets and the refrigerator. That way they are stored safely from insects, most pathogens, and the migration of toxic chemicals, e.g., BPA in plastic. There is plastic wrap [Whole Foods 365 brand Plastic Wrap] that contains no polyvinyl chloride (PVC), phthalates or Bisphenol A (BPA).

Also, it may be a good idea to check out and understand the numbering system within the triangle on the bottom of plastic food containers. Here's how to know what's safe. Visit online <ecovillagegreen.com/1812/ what-are-safe-plastic-numbers-to-use/>.

Aluminum-free Baking Powder Substitute

If you cannot find aluminum-free baking powder—some of which contain cornstarch, which can be from GMO corn, you can make an aluminum-free leavening agent at home by combining two ingredients: *Cream of Tartar and Baking Soda*. That is what I use. It gives great lift.

———

Here's the conversion rate that's equivalent to one (1) teaspoon of baking powder:

5/8 teaspoon Cream of Tartar AND
¼ teaspoon Baking Soda mixed together.

In the Organic Corn Bread recipe that follows, 4 teaspoons of aluminum-free baking powder are called for. To convert that into a homemade leavening agent, combine

2 ½ teaspoons Cream of Tartar with 1 teaspoon Baking Soda

It leaves no after-taste in the finished product, as there sometimes can be with baking powder. Commercial baking powders use chemicals—read the labels—for the acid/alkaline rising action.

Regarding Food Allergies

Again, I must remind you that it is important *NOT* to eat any foods to which you have food allergies as doing that places strain on the immune system which, of course, you want to avoid, as you are trying to build up and enhance an already compromised immune system.

Possible Clues to Food Allergies

Allergic food reactions can occur from immediately, which can be anaphylactic life-threatening and requires 911 services, up to 24 to 32 hours later depending upon *YOUR* body's chemistry.

Example:

Peanuts cause serious allergic reactions in many people, especially children, ranging from anaphylactic response to less severe.

Possible Other Allergic Reactions

Hives, which can appear within less than 30 minutes up to 24 hours; sweating; shaking; nervousness; agitation; rapid pulse; brain fog; diarrhea usually an hour or up to several hours later; dark circles under or around the eyes, referred to as "allergy shiners"; bloating of the abdomen; gripe-like intestinal pain and grumbling [2 or more hours after eating]; plus others that may be specific to *your* body chemistry.

Grain gluten is notorious for causing intestinal reactions. Soy also is an unsuspected reactionary food. When I studied nutrition I learned there could be a thousand allergic-type reactions in the human body from various challenges, as everyone's biochemistry though similar, differs slightly due to DNA, genetics, environment, and emotional input.

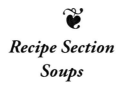

Recipe Section
Soups

Catherine's Special Nutrient-Rich Soup

[Makes 16 soup ladle servings]
Ingredients
1 cup organic *green* cabbage chopped
1 organic leek chopped
2 organic tomatoes chopped
3 organic garlic cloves put thru a garlic press
1 organic celery root (celeriac), cleaned, peeled, and chopped [if large, use half a root]
1 burdock root (brown, narrow and string-like) peeled and cut into coins
¼ teaspoon *Herbamare* (salt seasoning; health food store item)
1 ½ quarts/liters spring water, non-fluoridated
½ cup organic watercress leaves
¼ cup organic parsley chopped OR
1/8 cup cilantro for a different flavor OR
1/8 cup fresh dill for a different flavor
Bunch of scallions cleaned and chopped

Method
Combine all ingredients *except watercress, parsley, cilantro, dill, and scallions* into a large pot with lid.
Bring to boil; turn down heat to very low; place lid on.
Simmer 45 minutes.
Remove from heat and add watercress, parsley, scallions, and optional fresh herbs, e.g., cilantro or dill

Note: *When reheating the soup, never boil it. Allow the watercress, parsley, cilantro, dill and scallions to remain as raw as possible.*

For Added Trace Mineral Nutritional Value: Sprinkle a little dulse seaweed (similar to using salt) on top of a bowl or cup of soup when served. Add some raw sprouts as a topping to each bowl of soup, if you like.

Gazpacho [Spanish style cold soup] [4-8 servings]
Ingredients
  1 organic cucumber, peeled and sliced
  ½ organic sweet red pepper, sliced
  1 28 oz can organic whole tomatoes [BPA-free can]
  2 cloves organic garlic put thru garlic press
  1 organic lemon juiced
  2 Tablespoons organic olive oil
  ¼ teaspoon *Herbamare*
  Organic Cayenne pepper to taste

Method
  Into a blender cup layer ingredients this way for easy processing:
  cucumber, red pepper, tomatoes
  Process until blended
  Then add garlic, lemon juice, olive oil, *Herbamare,* and Cayenne pepper.
  Blend for about 25 seconds.

Transfer to large glass jar and refrigerate.
Always serve cold.

Non-Dairy Cream of Asparagus Soup

Ingredients

   2 lbs. fresh asparagus trimmed and cut into pieces
   1 large sweet (Vidalia type) onion chopped
   2 ribs celery chopped
   1 scant Tablespoon extra virgin olive oil
   1 Tablespoon fresh dill chopped (or ½ teaspoon dried dill)
   ½ teaspoon sea salt
   Cayenne pepper to taste
   1-½ liters spring water brought to a boil in a separate pot

Method

   Heat olive oil in a large pot with lid
   Add onions, asparagus, and celery
   Sauté vegetables until tender mixing often so as not to burn
   Add boiling water, dill, salt, and Cayenne pepper
   Turn heat to low; simmer 45 minutes with lid on pot
   Remove from heat and cool about 30 to 45 minutes or
until cool enough to place in a glass blender cup. Process each
batch about 15 seconds until creamy. Store in refrigerator in a
large ceramic bowl. Reheat but do not boil.

   Nutrition Note: Asparagus is an extremely rich source of
the antioxidant glutathione.

Vegetable Salad Recipes

Cucumber Salad
Ingredients
1 organic cucumber sliced
3 organic scallions sliced
¼ cup organic parsley chopped

Dressing
½ organic lemon juiced
1 Tablespoon organic olive oil
1 thin organic garlic clove put thru a garlic press
Combine all in a small bowl and whisk to blend.

Method
Combine all ingredients in a bowl and marinate a few hours in refrigerator.

Tomato Salad
1 organic Heirloom tomato sliced and placed on serving plate with rim to catch juices
Herbamare (salt seasoning)
Organic parsley chopped

Dressing
½ organic lemon juiced
1 Tablespoon organic olive oil
1 thin organic garlic clove put thru a garlic press

Combine all in a small bowl and whisk to blend.

Method

Arrange tomato slices on plate and sprinkle *Herbamare* on slices

Spoon ½ teaspoon dressing over each slice

Garnish generously with chopped parsley

Harvard Beet Salad

4 medium size organic red beets skins left on, scrubbed, leaves and 'tail' removed

Place beets on aluminum foil on the middle rack of a toaster oven and bake for 1 hr 15 minutes or a little longer at 425°F. Remove and allow to cool. Peel and dice into small pieces.

Dressing

½ large organic lemon juiced

1/8 teaspoon honey

scant amount of sea salt

Combine these ingredients into a small bowl and mix well until honey is blended in.

Add to diced beets. Mix well.

Drizzle ¼ teaspoon organic olive oil over beets and mix well.

Refrigerate. Eat as a side vegetable or as a topping on green salad.

Hijiki Seaweed Salad [8 servings]

Ingredients

1/8 cup *Hijiki* seaweed

1 teaspoon organic safflower oil smeared around to coat frying pan

¾ cup organic carrots, slivered or grated on large hole grater

½ sweet organic onion, thinly sliced

½ cup green beans cut French style (organic if possible)

1 ½ teaspoons organic soy sauce or organic *Tamari*

1 teaspoon honey

½ teaspoon fresh organic ginger finely grated

Organic Cayenne pepper to taste

1 teaspoon toasted sesame oil

Optional: Sprinkle with toasted sesame seeds

Method

Before beginning this recipe, soak seaweed in enough water to cover and set aside.

In a large frying pan or 10-inch skillet, heat safflower oil and sauté carrots, onion, and green beans for 3 minutes.

Drain seaweed and add to veggies.

Add soy sauce or *Tamari*, honey, ginger, and Cayenne pepper. Simmer 5 minutes.

Add toasted sesame oil, sesame seeds, and mix well. Refrigerate. Serve as vegetable or condiment with lunch or open face sandwiches.

The Perfect Green Salad

A green salad, in my opinion, is not Iceberg lettuce, grated carrots, and cherry tomatoes. Let's build a nutrient rich, *perfect* green salad, which should be made with organically grown greens and vegetables. Chlorophyll is a key nutrient in greens, which helps to cleanse and oxygenate the bloodstream. Just what a breast cancer patient needs, I think.

Greens—choose a selection of several from organically grown
Heirloom lettuces and greens
Romaine/Cos lettuce
Boston/Bibb lettuce
Frisée
Ruby Red or Green Loose Leaf lettuce
Oak Leaf lettuce
Spring Mix greens
Note: To see photographs of various lettuces and greens, please visit online <epicurious.com/articlesguides/seasonalcooking/farmtotable/visualguidesaladgreens>.

Toppings—choose a selection of several from organically grown
Arugula
Celeriac/celery root cut julienne or shoe string
Cucumber slices
Scallion rings
Sweet or red onion rings

Watercress leaves

Parsley leaves

Cilantro leaves

Leafy green sprouts like Arugula, broccoli, or mixed micro greens

Serve sliced organic tomato as a side vegetable on the dinner plate

Carrots contain too much sugar, so leave them out for now

Don't forget dried pumpkin seeds for added crunch instead of croutons

If you want to home-grow your own sprouts—make certain you use non-GMO seeds. You may want to check out this supplier on the web

<wheatgrasskits.com/sproutingkits.htm?gclid=CNyO2Jelo KwCFUKo4AodFUPs3Q>.

Dressings

Sorry, *NO* bottled or vinegar-type salad dressings, mayonnaise, mustard, sauces, and condiments. Use either fresh lemons or limes juiced for any recipe that you could convert that originally uses vinegar or salad dressing. Use red Cayenne pepper, which is an aide to digestion, instead of black pepper, which is hard to digest for some folks.

My Favorite Dressing

Juice of half a lemon, or my preference—half a lime, a little sea salt and organic extra virgin olive oil, plus a dash of Cayenne pepper.

Micro Green and Sprout Salad
You probably never heard of a salad like this. Being an innovative cook who had my own cooking show on TV (1980s) and having been a cooking instructor during my career, I devised what has become a favorite raw green salad, at least for me.

Ingredients
Organic pea sprout leaves on short stems
Organic mixed micro greens
Organic Arugula sprouts
Organic cherry tomatoes (Heirlooms preferred)
Juice of ½ lime
Herbamare and Cayenne pepper to taste
Drizzle of organic olive oil

Method
Arrange pea sprouts on a flat luncheon size plate
Add micro greens and Arugula sprouts
Slice cherry tomatoes and arrange on top of sprouts
Sprinkle with limejuice, *Herbamare*, and Cayenne pepper
Drizzle with organic olive oil.

What do you think?

Dip and Spread Recipes

Eggplant Dip/Pâté [Baba Ganoush] [4-8 servings]

Ingredients

1 organic eggplant washed and pricked with a fork in several places

1 organic lemon, juiced (only half a lemon if smaller eggplant)

2 cloves organic garlic put thru garlic press

2 heaping Tablespoons organic *Tahini* (sesame butter)

¼ teaspoon *Herbamare* (salt seasoning)

a little extra sea salt if desired

Cayenne pepper to taste, if desired

Method

Bake prepped eggplant on aluminum foil-lined oven rack at 400° for about 1 hr to 1 hr 15 minutes, depending upon size, or until soft and shriveled. Remove and let cool.

Peel off skin and place eggplant pulp into blender cup along with the rest of the ingredients.

Blend until smooth.

Transfer to a bowl or crock and refrigerate.

To Serve

Serve as a dressing for cooked vegetables: asparagus, broccoli, cauliflower, kale.

Serve as a generous open face sandwich spread on *one* slice of sourdough whole grain or yeast-free *Prairie Brown* bread with a slice of organic *Heirloom* tomato and topped with organic watercress leaves or sprouts

---

Serve as a dip for raw vegetables

Serve as a spread for a few yeast-free whole grain crackers or rice cake topped with sprouts as a snack

Hummus / Chick Pea Spread

Use the same recipe and method for *Eggplant Dip* above but with this exception:

One 15 oz can (*Eden* brand is BPA free) organic garbanzo beans (chick peas) drained and placed into a blender cup with enough of the can liquid to come only half-way up the beans in the blender cup.

Process a little then follow the above recipe to finish preparation. Same serving ideas apply to Hummus as with the Eggplant Dip.

Guacamole / Avocado spread/dip

Ingredients

1 ripe organic avocado

Juice of ½ organic lemon

2 small cloves organic garlic put thru garlic press

Sea salt to taste

Organic Cayenne pepper to taste

Method

Cut avocado in half; discard pit and peel

Place avocado into a shallow soup bowl; sprinkle with lemon juice

Mash finely using a fork

Add garlic, salt, and Cayenne pepper. Continue mashing with fork until creamy.

To Serve
- Sandwich spread on one piece of yeast-free bread open-face style with sliced tomato, cucumber, onion, salad greens, and sprouts
- Stuffing for Tacos or Tortillas
- Instead of butter as topping for a very small baked potato

Do NOT eat Guacamole with corn chips as you would normally. Here's the reason for my saying that: You will eat too many high starch carbohydrates in the chips.

Vegetable Dishes

Broccoli Italian style
Ingredients
    1 stalk broccoli cut into florets
    2-3 cloves organic garlic cloves sliced thinly
    1 teaspoon organic olive oil
    Herbamare to taste
    Cayenne pepper to taste

Method
    Clean, prep, and rinse broccoli. Place into a medium size fry pan with enough water to cover three-quarters. Bring to

boil, turn down heat to medium low, put lid on and simmer about 4 minutes. Remove lid, add garlic slices, turn up heat and cook until water is gone.

Remove from heat; add olive oil, *Herbamare*, and Cayenne pepper.

Special Cancer-fighting Nutrition Note: *Broccoli contains indol-3-carbinol, a powerful anti-carcinogen and antioxidant, beta-carotene (provitamin A), selenium, and zinc, which boost the immune system.*

Brussels sprouts, Best Ever in my opinion
Ingredients
20 *small* and sweet tasting Brussels sprouts cleaned of any damaged leaves with stem ends removed
½ teaspoon organic olive oil
Sprinkling of sea salt or *Herbamare*

Method
Place sprouts into a pot with a lid; add enough water to just about cover the sprouts.

Bring to boil, turn down heat to medium, cover with lid, and cook until water is gone.

Sprouts should be tender.

Add olive oil, and sea salt or *Herbamare*. Mix to cover all with seasonings.

Carrots Steamed with Tarragon

Ingredients

   2 medium size organic carrots peeled and cut into coins
   Organic olive oil, very light sprinkling
   Organic tarragon, very light sprinkling
   Herbamare sprinkling

Method

   Place sliced carrots into a pot with lid and cover with water. Bring to boil, turn down to simmer for 5 minutes, remove lid and allow water to cook out.

   Sprinkle olive oil, tarragon, and *Herbamare*. Serve hot or cold.

   Note: Even though carrots make a great snack or veggie with lunch, don't eat too many because of the sugars they contain.

Cauliflower Quick and Delicious

Ingredients

   1 cup organic cauliflower florets
   ¼ teaspoon organic olive oil
   Herbamare sprinkling
   Organic dill weed sprinkling
   Organic Cayenne pepper sprinkling

Method

   Pare any black marks [fungus usually] from cauliflower and place into pot with lid.

Add enough water to cover cauliflower half way; bring to boil; turn heat down to medium; place lid on pot; and check for tenderness. Drain water and drink as tea. Add olive oil, *Herbamare*, dill weed, and Cayenne pepper.

Other Vegetables Quick and Delicious

Asparagus, Bok Choy, Broccoli Rabe (Rappini), shredded cabbage, collard greens, and spinach can be prepared and cooked lightly using the same method in the recipes for Broccoli Italian Style and Cauliflower. It's quick, easy, and nutritious.

Cauliflower Stew [2 servings]
Ingredients
   ½ head organic cauliflower chopped
   1 organic sweet onion chopped
   1 rib organic celery chopped
   1 small/thin organic carrot chopped
   1 teaspoon organic curry powder
   ½ teaspoon organic turmeric
   ¼ teaspoon *Herbamare* (salt seasoning)
   Non-fluoridated spring water to cover chopped veggies
   ½ cup frozen baby peas
   3 Tablespoons slivered almonds

Optional to make thick gravy
   1 ½ teaspoons *organic* non-GMO cornstarch
   1 teaspoon water

Combine in small bowl to make a slurry to thicken stew

Method

In a large 10-inch skillet or fry pan combine all ingredients *except* peas, almonds, and cornstarch.

Cover with water and cook for about 10 minutes until cauliflower is tender.

Add cornstarch slurry to thicken stew; add frozen peas and almonds, and cook for about 3 minutes longer to cook off cornstarch taste.

To Serve

Spoon heaping Tablespoons of Cauliflower Stew over a small amount of either cooked brown rice or mashed potatoes. Serve with large green salad and Daikon radish.

Leftover Stew

Make a 2-organic-egg omelet. Have stew heated in separate pan. Spoon stew onto omelet, fold over and serve as a delicious entrée with a steamed vegetable and green salad.

Special Cancer-fighting Nutrition Note: *Cauliflower contains beta-carotene (provitamin A) and phytonutrients that protect against free radicals; sulforaphane and indole-3-carbinol, cancer-fighting agents; and Omega-3 fatty acids.*

Green Beans Italian style

Ingredients

¼ lb green beans [string beans] ends trimmed

2-3 cloves organic garlic sliced thinly

½ teaspoon organic olive oil

Herbamare to taste

Cayenne pepper to taste

Method

Clean, prep, and rinse green beans. Place into a medium size fry pan with enough water to cover. Bring to boil, turn down heat to medium, put lid on and simmer until water is half gone. Remove lid, add garlic slices, and cook until water is gone.

Remove from heat; add olive oil, *Herbamare*, and Cayenne pepper.

Note: **Fresh spinach** can be prepared using the green bean recipe above. There is only one exception to the recipe: Very little water, enough to cover the bottom of the pan because you will be turning the spinach and garlic often to cook just 'til tender about 1-2 minutes, otherwise the spinach tastes bitter the longer it cooks. Take off heat and add olive oil, *Herbamare*, and Cayenne pepper.

Sweet Red Pepper Sauté

Ingredients

1 large organic sweet red pepper sliced

1 medium organic sweet onion sliced

3 cloves organic garlic cloves sliced

1 Tablespoon organic olive oil

Sea salt and Cayenne pepper to taste

Method

Coat the bottom of a large stainless steel fry pan with olive oil and heat.

Add sweet red peppers, onions, garlic, salt and Cayenne pepper.

Using a wooden spoon or wooden fork, mix constantly over medium heat to prevent caramelizing and/or scorching or burning.

When vegetables are limp, about 5 minutes, remove from pan and serve either hot as a side vegetable or cold leftovers on top of salad greens or in sandwich wraps.

Zucchini Sauté [2 servings]
Ingredients

1 medium organic zucchini cut into large chunks [slice lengthwise two times to make 4 sections, then cut those sections into 1 inch cubes]

½ organic sweet onion chopped

1 large organic tomato chopped

2 cloves organic garlic chopped

Sprinkling of organic dried basil

Sprinkling of sea salt and Cayenne pepper to taste

½ teaspoon organic olive oil

Juice of ½ lime

Method

Coat the bottom of a large fry pan with olive oil, tilting to spread oil around.

Place onions, zucchini, and tomato into pan in that order. Shake pan to coat veggies. Turn heat to medium and stir often.

Add garlic, basil, salt, Cayenne pepper, and lime juice.

Stir until zucchini is crunchy and serve.

Additional Serving Suggestion: Reheat leftovers and place over 1 slice of organic sourdough bread for a hot open-face sandwich topped with sprouts and served with a cup of soup and a salad.

Vegetable Stir-Fry

Ingredients

  ½ organic sweet onion chopped
  ½ organic sweet red pepper chopped
  ¾ cup organic broccoli spears
  6 organic asparagus chopped
  6 organic Bok Choy ribs with leaves chopped
  1 thin organic carrot sliced into coins
  4 cloves organic garlic sliced
  6 organic scallions sliced into coins
  ¼ cup diced organic celery root (celeriac)
  Optional: burdock root cut into coins

1 teaspoon fresh organic ginger peeled and grated finely

1 scant Tablespoon organic safflower oil

1 teaspoon organic Tamari sauce

organic red pepper flakes to taste (hot stuff)

½ teaspoon toasted sesame seed oil

Method

Clean, wash, prepare, slice, and dice all vegetables placing them in a strainer or colander.

Using a large 10-inch stainless steel fry pan [does the best job for stir-frying], coat the bottom with safflower oil and heat.

Add veggies in this order: onions, sweet red peppers, broccoli spears, carrots and burdock root [stirring constantly] cook 2 minutes, then add asparagus, Bok Choy, celery root, garlic, and stir fry for about 2 minutes.

Add Tamari sauce, ginger, scallions and stir-fry for another minute or two. Drizzle with sesame oil, mix well. Remove from heat and enjoy with small baked organic potato or organic quinoa, and raw organic green salad.

Quinoa Stuffed Zucchini Boats

Ingredients

Cook quinoa while preparing vegetables

½ cup organic quinoa (*red* preferred but others will do) thoroughly rinsed and placed into a pot with 1 cup spring water water. Bring to a boil, turn down to simmer, place lid on pot and cook 15 minutes. Remove lid and cook until water is gone.

2 6-8 inch long slender organic zucchinis cut in half lengthwise with insides scooped out, diced and set aside

¼ cup organic yellow sweet pepper diced

1 rib organic celery diced

6 organic scallions cut into coins

2 cloves organic garlic diced

1 Tablespoon fresh organic ginger diced

½ large organic lime juiced

1 Tablespoon organic olive oil

1/3 cup cooked quinoa

Salt OR *Herbamare* to taste

Optional: a few cilantro leaves chopped

Method

Make certain quinoa is dry and fluffy like cooked rice

Heat a fry pan with olive oil; add all chopped veggies except scallions and cilantro

Sauté veggies on medium heat for about 5 minutes

Add quinoa, scallions, and cilantro

Remove from heat, add limejuice and mix thoroughly

Stuff zucchini shells with mixture and arrange in large baking dish (9" pie pan will do)

Add water half way up the sides of zucchini boats and bake in 375°F oven 45 minutes

Boats will be crunchy but delicious

Leftover Quinoa

Eat left over quinoa as a breakfast cereal either heated or cold with almond or coconut milk. Add a few chopped organic English walnuts for extra nutrition and crunch.

Egg Frittatas

First and foremost, I recognize that food purist *aficionados* reading this book may be upset about cooking eggs with the yolks scrambled, which I don't recommend as a prime way for cooking eggs, e.g., scrambled eggs. However, these two frittata recipes offer an entrée that works nicely for dinner with any leftovers served cold, diced on a salad or as an open face sandwich with plenty of sprouts, sliced tomatoes, and green lettuce.

Potato-Onion Egg Frittata [1 serving]

1 very *small* organic Red Bliss potato peeled and thinly sliced; use potato peeler to make slices

½ organic sweet onion thinly sliced

1 Tablespoon organic olive oil

Sprinkling of *Herbamare*

1 organic egg

1 organic *egg white only*

Method

In an 8-inch stainless steel fry pan, heat oil and when hot, add potatoes, onions, and *Herbamare*. Turn heat to medium and stir constantly for about 4 minutes until potatoes are tender. Set aside.

Beat eggs in a separate bowl.

Use olive oil to grease an 8-inch baking dish or ovenproof fry pan (Corning brand is good). Pour in eggs and then add the potato-onion mixture. Mix with fork to distribute vegetables evenly.

Bake in a 350°F oven about 10-12 minutes, depending upon how quickly the eggs set.

Use a spatula to remove the frittata and serve as an entrée with steamed green veggies, e.g., asparagus and broccoli, or green beans and kale, or green beans Italiano, or spinach, together with either cucumber salad or tomato salad and green salad. *No bread!* The potato has enough carbs.

Zucchini Frittata [1 serving]

1 small thin organic zucchini, grated on the large hole of a hand grater

½ organic sweet onion thinly sliced

1 Tablespoon organic olive oil

Sprinkling of *Herbamare*

Several sprinklings organic dried dill weed

1 organic egg

1 organic *egg white only*

Method

In an 8-inch stainless steel fry pan, heat oil and when hot, add zucchini, onions, *Herbamare,* and dill weed. Turn heat to medium and stir constantly for about 2-3 minutes until veggies are tender. Set aside.

Beat eggs in a separate bowl.

Use olive oil to grease an 8-inch baking dish or ovenproof fry pan (Corning brand is good). Pour in eggs and then add the zucchini-onion mixture. Mix with fork to distribute zucchini evenly.

Bake in a 350°F oven about 10-12 minutes, depending upon how quickly the eggs set.

Use a spatula to remove the frittata and serve as an entrée with steamed green veggies, e.g., Broccoli Rabe and Bok Choy, **OR** green beans and kale, together with either cucumber salad or tomato salad and green salad. *One slice* of organic sourdough, yeast-free whole grain bread may be eaten with this.

Haricots Vert (French Green Beans)

Very thin string beans that steam up in 3 to 4 minutes. Serve leftovers cold with salad.

Beans, Legumes, and Grains

Garbanzo Bean Stew

Ingredients

1 15 oz can organic garbanzo beans (chickpeas) drained (*Eden* brand BPA-free cans)

1 organic sweet onion chopped coarsely

1 organic red potato, skin scrubbed (not peeled) and chopped coarsely

2 ribs organic celery chopped coarsely

1 ripe organic tomato chopped

1 thin organic carrot chopped coarsely

½ teaspoon organic or non-irradiated curry powder (*Frontier* brand)

½ teaspoon sea salt

½ teaspoon fresh organic ginger grated finely

1 clove organic garlic put thru a garlic press

2 pods cardamom (smash pods to remove seeds for stew) (*Frontier* brand)

1 thin organic zucchini chopped coarsely

Method

Into a large heavy pot with a lid, place the onion, potato, celery, tomato, and carrot with enough pure water to cover.

Bring to a boil; turn down heat to a medium slow simmer.

Add garbanzo beans, curry powder, salt, ginger, garlic, and cardamom seeds. Cook stew 45 minutes on medium slow simmer with lid on pot, stirring occasionally.

Then add zucchini and cook on medium slow simmer for 10 additional minutes.

To Serve

This is a hearty stew that tastes even better the next day. However, this stew should be eaten with a large green salad and another green vegetable, e.g., asparagus, to balance out the starchy carbohydrates. This makes a wonderfully satisfying winter night's dinner. When eaten as suggested, this stew can make three meals for one person.

Note: No other carbohydrates with this meal; the beans, potato, and carrot are plenty.

Gently Spiced Lentils
Ingredients
    ½ cup organic lentils picked over to make certain there are no stones and rinsed
    2 cloves organic garlic put thru garlic press
    ½ organic sweet onion finely chopped
    1 ½ cups spring water
    ½ teaspoon grated fresh organic ginger
    ¼ teaspoon *Herbamare*
    ¼ teaspoon organic turmeric
    Sprinkling of organic cinnamon
    ½ teaspoon honey

Method
    Place all ingredients into a medium size pot with a lid.
    Bring to a boil; turn heat down to low; place lid on pot; and cook for 1 hour or until lentils are soft. May need to add a little water toward the end. Stir several times during cooking.

    To Serve: Consider lentils to be similar to a serving of meat. Add plenty of green vegetables and green salad to complete a meal with lentils.

Organic Cornbread [8 servings]
Ingredients

1 cup organic *non-GMO* cornmeal [*Bob's Red Mill* is an organic brand]

1 cup organic whole grain spelt flour [*Bob's Red Mill* is an organic brand]

½ teaspoon sea salt

4 teaspoons aluminum-free baking powder [*Rumford* brand] (*or substitute 2 ½ teaspoons Cream of Tartar and 1 teaspoon baking soda, which equals 4 teaspoons baking powder*)

1 organic egg

1 cup organic light coconut milk

2 Tablespoons *honey* definitely NO table sugar

4 Tablespoons organic olive oil

2 teaspoons organic vanilla extract

Method

Preheat oven to 375°F and grease an 8"x 8" baking dish with olive oil.

To grease baking pan: Pour a few drops of olive oil into baking pan and spread around with a paper towel, making certain to get into the corners and up the sides of pan.

Combine dry ingredients in large bowl and mix well.

Combine beaten egg, coconut milk, honey, olive oil, and vanilla in another bowl. Mix well to blend all liquid ingredients.

Add liquid ingredients to dry ingredients.

Mix until smooth, or about 1 minute. **Don't over beat or over mix.**

Pour into greased baking pan and bake 25 minutes in 400ºF oven or until tester comes out clean.

To Serve

Slightly warm with *no-sugar* pure fruit jam. (St. Dalfour Spreads from France are made *without* cane sugar and only four ingredients: fruit, grape juice, fruit pectin, and lemon juice. Unfortunately, organically grown USA fruit spreads contain organic cane sugar, which I do not consider healthful in diets dealing with breast cancer.)

Suggestion: Cut corn bread into 8 sections/slices and freeze each section separately in wax paper stored in a freezer bag in the freezer. Take out a piece to defrost and eat as needed. Cornbread pieces can be warmed up in a toaster oven at 250ºF for about 2-3 minutes.

Almond-Cornbread for a different taste treat

Use and follow the above recipe with this exception instead of 1 cup cornmeal:

¼ cup Almond Meal/Flour *[Bob's Red Mill brand—note the almond meal is not organic]*

¾ cup organic *non-GMO* cornmeal *[Bob's Red Mill* is an organic brand]

NEVER eat the entire cornbread in one sitting. It's tempting, though! **Too many carbs.**

———

Quinoa

This South American grain—actually a seed—is packed with lignans and phytonutrients that are important in reducing cancer risks. Quinoa is high in *vegetable* protein, about 16 percent per volume. Purchase organically grown Quinoa, which usually comes from South America.

Prepare quinoa according to package instructions and eat as morning cereal with coconut or almond milk, or prepare a quinoa salad with chopped onions or scallions, cherry tomatoes, chopped celery, small amount of diced raw zucchini, loads of chopped parsley, 1 clove of garlic put thru a garlic press, and tossed with lemon juice, olive oil, salt, and Cayenne pepper. Use organically grown veggies. Refrigerate and eat like potato salad.

Vegetarian Quinoa "Paella"
Prepare Quinoa

½ cup organic red quinoa (better taste than other colors, I think) rinsed well and cooked in one cup pure water for 15 minutes on medium heat with lid on the pot. When cooked, it resembles cooked rice. While quinoa is cooking, prepare vegetables.

Ingredients
   1 Tablespoon organic olive oil
   ½ cup organic red cabbage chopped
   ½ organic sweet red pepper chopped

3 ribs organic celery chopped

1 organic sweet onion chopped

½ contents of 28oz can whole organic tomatoes (BPA free can); cut tomatoes into chunks

2 cloves garlic chopped

¼ teaspoon *Herbamare*

Slight sprinkling of sea salt

1/8 teaspoon dried organic dill weed

Method

Heat olive oil in a large 10-inch, fry pan.

Add all chopped vegetables except tomatoes, *Herbamare*, and sea salt.

Sauté about 5 minutes on medium heat.

Add tomatoes cut into chunks.

Mix well, then add dill weed and

4 heaping Tablespoons cooked red quinoa

Mix well and turn heat to very low. Place lid on fry pan and cook about 3 minutes.

Pardon my saying this, but this quinoa recipe is so delicious, you will go back for seconds. Serve with a *Perfect Green Salad* and *Cucumber Salad*.

Note: Any cooked red quinoa not used in the recipe can be served as breakfast cereal.

Desserts

Stewed Apples
2 organic apples scrubbed, skins left on, and cut into large chunks

Place into a pot with enough water to come ¾ way up the apples.

Bring to a boil, turn down to simmer until chunky, not mushy.

Baked Apples
2 organic apples scrubbed and cored, leave skins on
Sprinkle inside core with some organic cinnamon.
Stuff core with organic walnut pieces.
Place in baking pan (pie pan will do) with 1 cup of water.
Bake 45 minutes to 1 hour in a 375°F oven. Occasionally baste apples with pan water.
Can be served warm or cold, plain or with coconut milk.

Pumpkin Custard Pudding
This recipe makes six decadently delicious pumpkin custard ramekins tasting like pumpkin pie but without the crust and flour.
1 15 oz can organic pumpkin
1 cup organic light coconut milk (I use pure water sometimes or half water and half coconut milk)
2 large organic eggs beaten
2 Tablespoons orange blossom *or* clover honey
2 teaspoons organic vanilla
½ teaspoon organic *Pumpkin Pie Spice Blend* (*Frontier* brand)

½ teaspoon organic cinnamon
¼ teaspoon sea salt

Method

Place pumpkin into a large mixing bowl with spice blend, cinnamon, and salt. Mix well.

In another bowl combine coconut milk (water), eggs, honey, and vanilla mixing well to dissolve honey.

Add liquid to pumpkin and using a wire whisk, mix until blended very well, as mixture is thick.

Ladle into 6 individual one-ladle size, ovenproof ramekins placed in a baking pan with about ¾ inch of warm water.

Bake in 375°F oven 45 minutes. This will be a soft custard, but oh so special.

Refrigerate and eat as dessert or snack topped with chopped organic walnuts.

Note: I have a friend who, when he eats this, shuts his eyes and moans. I've asked why and the answer is "*so good.*"

Special Cancer-fighting Nutrition Note: Pumpkin contains *phytosterols*, which may be effective in preventing cancer; *zinc,* which boosts the immune system and promotes healing; and *tryptophan* that helps in dealing with depression.

Mock Eggnog

While writing this book, Thanksgiving was fast approaching. Being an innovative and creative cook—I had my own TV cooking show, *Catherine's Natural Kitchen,* and taught natural-style cooking classes in my own 'school' and as a guest cook for other 'schools', I wondered what could those folks drink who want to 'imbibe' during the holidays. While making my cornbread recipe, I came up with the following concoction, which I think really puts one in mind of Eggnog, but without the 'kick' and sugar. See what you think.

1 can organic light coconut milk (can be cut with some water)
1 teaspoon organic liquid vanilla
1 ½ teaspoons clover honey
Organic ground nutmeg, a pinch or two

Method
Shake coconut milk can very well to mix the contents, then empty it into a large bowl.

Add vanilla (water), honey, and nutmeg making certain to mix very well so that honey is incorporated into the liquid. I recommend using a wire whisk or a stick blender. At this point, taste and see how it sits with your taste buds. If a tad bit of honey is needed, add it, but be careful because if the recovering cancer patient is going to drink it, there may be too much sugar content from the honey.

For the recipes in this book, the only sweetener I use and the body can handle much more efficiently and *on rare occasion for the cancer patient*, is *pure* honey.

How to check if honey is adulterated and not pure bee honey

Into a glass of water drop half-a-teaspoonful of honey. If it dissolves immediately, it's NOT pure/real honey. Pure/real honey stays in a glob state and has to be mixed thoroughly to dissolve.

Much of the honey sold in grocery stores contains more than bee-produced honey sweeteners. I recommend purchasing local beekeeper honey. However, if you know for certain that your health food store sells only 100 percent pure honey, not imported 'honey', go for it. See this Internet website for more information about adulterated honey <foodsafetynews.com/2011/08/honey-laundering/>.

Piña Colada

The above *Mock Eggnog* recipe can be used to make a *Piña Colada* by adding ¼ to ½ cup of canned pineapple juice and omitting the nutmeg. Forget the rum, if you want to serve it to kiddies as a holiday time drink. This recipe would not be suitable for the recovering cancer patient because of the fruit juice and honey (and rum, if added) too much sugar that will entice candida growth, which we want to keep from getting out of control, and not feed nor fertilize cancer cells.

Note: These are some ideas for recipes that keep the diet and food intake targeting both body pH plus optimum nutrient content and, of course, as yeast-free and non-candida inducing as possible.

May I suggest for more exciting yeast-free recipes, your checking out *THE YEAST-FREE KITCHEN, Recipes To Help You Achieve Victory Over The Yeast-Beast: Candida Albicans*, by Jane Remington, ISBN 141200797-6 (available on Amazon. com).

Jane is a cancer survivor for many years now, who has a passion for helping others overcome that disease. Additionally, Jane is a *fabulous* gourmet cook who has created exceptional recipes that not only are delicious, yeast-free, but oh so easy to make. Jane includes meat and fish recipes in her cookbook. However, I'm of the persuasion that the more vegetarian one can become with diet, the better the results will be. Dr Max Gerson proved that a long time ago.

Thin-skin onions predict a mild winter, thick-skin onions, a very tough one!

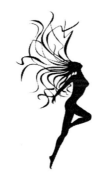

Chapter Twenty-One
Cancer Management Diets

Don't dig your grave with your own knife and fork.

… English Proverb

There are numerous diets that have gained notoriety for managing cancer. Below is a listing for Internet websites to obtain more information about them. Personally for me, the diet I maintained during my odyssey has worked extremely well in providing the nutrients needed to '*ungrow*' a large mass of two tumors in my right breast. As of April 2012, my right breast looks like my left breast, no tumor protrusion that was the size of half a large orange. There are neither incision marks nor radiation exposure burns, for which I am extremely grateful.

Each breast cancer patient has to find what works best for her—or him. However, I'd like to caution that if you continue eating a diet that is based in fast food, processed foods, unhealthful fats, dairy, and red meats, I don't think your body will respond and be able to work with you to heal your condition. I say that from my education, having been in practice as a consulting *natural* nutritionist, and now my own experience.

All diets listed below have several things in common: tremendous amounts of vegetables and raw foods, salads, vegetable juices; NO sugars and sweeteners nor foods made with them, and definitely NO genetically modified organisms (GMOs).

Budwig Diet   <cancure.org/budwig_diet.htm>
The Budwig Cancer & Coronary Heart Disease Prevention Diet: The Revolutionary Diet from Dr. Johanna Budwig is the book written by the researcher who discovered Omega-3 fatty acids. Her book is available on Amazon.com.

Dr Kelly's Metabolic Cancer Cure Diet
<educate-yourself.org/cancer/kellymetabolicdiet13dec02.shtml>

Gerson Therapy Diet   <gerson.org>
Juicing and raw foods diet

Macrobiotic Diet / The Kushi Institute
<kushiinstitute.org/waytohealth/macrobiotics/moreinfo.htm>

Organic Food Store Locator

Some breast cancer patients may not live near organic style supermarkets, co-ops, etc. Organic foods are available anywhere in the USA. I've provided an online locator for organic foods. An easy way to find Organic Food Stores in all 50 states in the USA is available online at <organicstorelocator.com/>.

Food—not money—just may be the root of many evils.

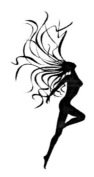

Chapter Twenty-Two
Antioxidants, Free Radicals, and Exercise

It is virtually impossible to get the optimal amount of
antioxidants through food alone.

… Lester Packer, PhD
Foremost antioxidant research scientist

*D*r Lester Packer is the foremost researcher and author about every aspect of antioxidants and human health. He has published over 800 scientific papers and 100 books on the subject.

What is an antioxidant?

Basically, an antioxidant is a substance that protects cells against and from the damage of free radicals, which are products of oxidation that attack healthy cells. There's a definite link between chronic overproduction of free radicals and disease in the human body, particularly with regard to inflammatory-related diseases and chronic disease patterns. Cancer is one disease that finds part of its genesis in free radical production. Other factors include genetics/heredity estimated at less than 10 percent, chemical exposure, imprudent/bad lifestyle habits, and aging—just getting old.

> *Cigarette smoking is the most potent free radical generator in the body. Even one or two puffs sends the amount of oxidative stress on your body soaring. Environmental pollution, fried foods and charcoal broiled meats also increase oxidative stress,* according to Bill Salt, MD, in answer to the question, "What causes free radicals in the body?" [97]

So, your lifestyle, together with diet and eating habits, definitely need to be assessed and changed in order *to stop and prevent* as much free radical production as possible in your body. Free radicals naturally occur in the body as a result of normal life processes, especially those involving the digestion of food. However, really bad habits like smoking and eating an unhealthful diet of junk, charbroiled, fried, and fast foods, which contribute inordinate amounts of free radicals, must be discontinued to overcome cancer.

If you happen to be hooked on soda, then you need to understand the role it plays in free radical production within your body. High levels of phosphorus alone in soda are associated with the aging process, thereby inducing greater free radical production. I suggest checking out information as to why you should refrain from drinking soda. *Science Daily* put together a great exposé about phosphate in soda in its online article "Early Death by Junk Food? High Levels of Phosphate in Sodas and Processed Foods Accelerate the Aging Process in Mice." You may want to read that article a few times to understand why you have to give up soda, and finally believe. That article can be found online at <sciencedaily.com/releases/2010/04/100426151636.htm>.

If you have been exposed to toxic chemicals either at work or home—via pesticides, tobacco smoke, household cleaning products, hazardous materials, etc.—your body most likely is harboring toxins. If there are toxic metals in your body, e.g., aluminum, mercury [ingredients in most vaccines [98]] arsenic, cadmium, lead, etc., even essential minerals like copper and iron can attain toxic overloads, your body will have higher amounts of free radicals.

A key aspect of antioxidants is their ability to force oxygen into aerobic pathways.

Detoxification is a crucial modality for eliminating both heavy metals and free radical production. A hair test can reveal which toxic metals are stored in your body. There are numerous programs under the care and direction of a physician to detoxify toxic metals, either orally or via chelation that use various chelating agents, e.g., Dimercaprol, Dimercaptosuccinic acid, Dimercapto-propane sulfonate, Penicillamine, Ethylenediamine tetraacetic acid (EDTA), Deferoxamine, and Deferasirox, etc.

For more information about chelation therapy—usually done by allopathic MDs to detoxify for lead—may I suggest visiting *Wikipedia* online at <en.wikipedia.org/wiki/Chelation_therapy>.

Alpha Lipoic Acid (ALA) is a supplement form of chelating agent.

Free radicals damage DNA and that disrupts the normal production of cells, which then reproduce or replicate not according to inherited *healthy* genetic DNA information. Instead, free radicals induce weak, confused cancer cells whose reproductive processes differ from normal healthy cells. The main location for free radical damage in DNA is found within the mitochondria—the powerhouse—of cells.

Exercise

Cancer cells can't live, thrive, and multiply in a highly oxygenated body. Exercise is an excellent method for increasing oxygen delivery to cells—that's if you can exercise without getting tired or dragging you down.

One of the best exercises is walking at a fast pace for about 20 minutes in an area with plenty of trees, like a park. Never walk on a road where you will be forced to breathe automotive and diesel exhaust fumes thereby causing MORE free radical production.

Also practice deep breathing exercises. I suggest visiting these websites for learning the techniques of deep breathing:
- <buzzle.com/articles/basic-breathing-techniques.html>
- Dr Andrew Weil's three deep breathing techniques at <drweil.com/drw/u/ART00521/three-breathing-exercises.html>

- <pilates.about.com/od/pilateswarmupandprep/a/ breathingEx.htm>

Always remember: Never overdo it! Do only as much as you feel comfortable doing without getting tired, winded, or light headed.

Sources of Antioxidants

Antioxidants are found naturally in food, plus via nutritional supplements. The more processed your food is, the lesser quality of antioxidants may be found because of *antioxidant damage* from heat, evaporation, storage, food processing, or chemicals.

Naturally occurring food sources of antioxidants are foods high in vitamins A and beta-carotene, vitamins C and E. *All berries are rich in antioxidants.* However, chocolate should not be considered an antioxidant, in my opinion. When I studied nutrition I learned that chocolate destroys many of the water-soluble B vitamins in the body—for whatever that may be worth.

Broccoli, Brussels sprouts, carrots, and tomatoes are exceptional sources of antioxidants.

Organic *whole* grains, e.g., brown rice, *whole* wheat, spelt, are rich sources of vitamin E, another antioxidant. See Chapter 19, *Foods HIGH in Sulfur,* for more information.

Another form of antioxidants that you may want to consider and discuss with your health professional is an antioxidant in supplement [pill] form. Between an antioxidant-rich diet and nutritional supplements—I take several daily—your body ought to be able to overcome the damaging effects of free radicals and prevent further free radical damage to cells.

One company, *Vitamin Code,* produces a *Raw Antioxidants* formula that, in my professional opinion as a retired *natural nutritionist,* is extremely bioavailable since it is made with and from close to 100 percent organically-grown RAW ingredients—food sources, not petrochemicals made in a factory—that the body recognizes and can utilize with full efficiency, and not tax the liver and other organs of detoxification. Additionally, antioxidants strengthen the immune system by providing free radical intervention and protection.

Regarding antioxidants, I just happened to find these interesting quotes about them, which I think are most impressive and also explain why antioxidants are so important. I found them at *Dr Packer Quotes*[99] apparently referring to Lester Packer, PhD, and his book, *The Antioxidant Miracle,* published in 1999. [100]

"Although there are literally hundreds of antioxidants, only five appear to be network antioxidants: Vitamins C and E, glutathione, lipoic acid and Coenzyme Q10." - p. 9

"What makes network antioxidants so special is that they can recycle, or regenerate, one another after they have quenched a free radical." - p. 17

"The number of oxidative hits daily to DNA per human cell is about 10,000. Now multiply that by the trillions of cells in the body." - p. 18

"Lipoic acid is the most versatile and powerful antioxidant in the entire antioxidant defense network." - p. 19

Antioxidants in Supplement Form
The following is a listing of readily available
antioxidants in dry or gel capsule.
This is NOT a recommendation that you take them.
Please discuss your taking any supplements
with your healthcare professional.
Some MAY interfere with chemotherapy
and/or radiation, i.e.,
These agents include the anthracyclines *(eg, doxorubicin),*
platinum-containing complexes (eg, cisplatin, carboplatin),
alkylating agents (eg, cyclophosphamide, ifosfamide), and cyto-
toxic antibiotics (eg, bleomycin, mitomycin-C). [101]

Antioxidants

Acai Berry
Acetyl-L-Carnitine
Alpha Lipoic Acid
Astaxanthin

Beta Carotene
Bilberry
Catalase
Copper (as chelated mineral)
COQ-10 [the *trans-form* type (on the label) and not synthetic made from tobacco leaves]
Cysteine

Gingko
Glutathione
Grape Seed Extract
Green Tea Extract

Lutein
Lycopene
Manganese (as chelated mineral)
Milk Thistle

Olive leaf extract
Omega-3 Fatty Acids

Pycnogenol
Quercetin
Resveratrol

Seaweed
Selenium (as chelated mineral)
Superoxide Dismutase (SOD)
Turmeric / Curcumin

Vitamin A
Vitamin C
Vitamin E
Vitamin K_2

Zinc (as chelated mineral)

Antioxidants in Tea

In addition to the supplement form, antioxidants abound greatly in some teas, especially organic green tea with its *epigallocatechin gallate,* or EGCG. EGCG decreases the risk of metastasis and the production of *estradiol*—strongest *natural* form of estrogen—while providing protection against damaging effects of chemotherapy. Black teas have less EGCG because they are allowed to oxidize during processing. Some think that *Red Rooibos* tea, made from a South African herb, contains flavonoids found in green tea but no EGCG. However, statements are made that Rooibos contains antioxidants and, of course, that it is caffeine-free.

Interestingly, Lesley M Butler and Anna H Wu, authors of the paper "Green and black tea in relation to gynecologic cancers" published May 19, 2011 online in *Molecular Nutrition Food Research,* state that the green tea *catechin epigallocatechin-3-gallate* inhibits growth and induces apoptosis [cell suicide] in HPV infected cervical cells and in cervical cancer cells. However, in another paper, "Green tea and breast cancer," those same authors concluded green tea's role in breast cancer still is not clear because of the paucity of epidemiological studies on green tea and breast cancers.

I consider myself a connoisseur or maven regarding teas, especially green teas—*Gunpowder Green* and *Jasmine Green* vie for being my favorites. Here's some information I'd like to pass along, especially for my readers who brew their tea using tea bags.

Please consider that many tea bags are bleached and also contain chemicals such as *epichlorohydrin, a compound used in the manufacture of plastics and used as an insecticide. When this chemical comes into contact with water it forms a chemical called 3-MCPD, a known cancer causing agent.* [102]

Please keep in mind that boiling water poured over chemical-laden tea bags constitutes a whammy you just don't want to play with, in my opinion. Instead of obtaining the benefits of tea, you will be ingesting cancer-causing chemicals. One tea supplier whose teas I drink is *Choice Organic Teas.* They use only natural fiber, unbleached tea bags. [103]

I think I may be coming addicted to their *Jasmine Green and White Peony* teas. Another tea producer, the Bigelow Tea Company, says it does not use epichlorohydrin is their tea bags. Dr Kristie Leong, MD, discusses hidden dangers in tea bags in her article "The Hidden Health Risks of Tea Bags." [102]

Green tea also has a diuretic effect, which means more potty trips—something very important for clearing toxins and dead cancer cells. Don't be surprised if you find yourself saying, "Take tea and pee."

Eat right, get some exercise, think lovely thoughts, and definitely get enough rest.

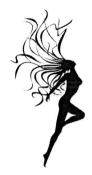

Chapter Twenty-Three
Water, Hydration, and The Lymphatic System

Water is the most neglected nutrient in your diet, but one of the most vital.

… **Julia Child (1912—2004)**
TV's French chef

*U*nlike most authors who discuss holistic cancer treatments, I will not talk about what usually is referred to as a "water cure." What I want to discuss, explain, and impress upon you is the important physiological role water plays in health: i.e., hydration of the body and cellular activity, viscosity of body fluids, nutrient transport, brain size and even cognitive ability, cellular waste transport and removal, and its impact upon the lymphatic system—most important for breast issues, any type of cancer, or disease in general.

To visualize lymphatics—part of the immune system—we should consider them almost as a 'drainage' system with two types of pressure that move fluids. There's the *hydrostatic pressure*, which is our blood pressure, and the counterbalancing *oncotic pressure* from blood proteins that are suspended in fluid. The give-and-take between both pressures is what keeps the body's tissues clean of various elements that can cause damage, especially free radical damage.

The lymph vessels also collect dead cells, waste products, bacteria, viruses, inorganic substances, water and fats. [104]

Since most of the water in our bodies is found within the lymph system, it's important to drink half your body weight in ounces daily to enable the body to detoxify. So how much water is that? If you weigh 150 pounds, you should be drinking 75 ounces of *pure* water a day, or 2 liters plus an 8 ounce glass of *pure* water. There are 33.8 ounces in a liter. Sodas, coffee, tea, and other beverages do not count as water.

Proper drainage of the lymphatic system is essential because that process enhances the immune system. Perhaps nothing contributes as effectively as *pure* water [H_2O]. So in keeping the lymphatic system humming along nicely, you can understand how important that becomes in view of the above statement in italics that showcases the vital work lymph vessels do for the body. We can help lymphatic drainage further by learning how to do a lymphatic massage or obtain a massage from a professionally trained massage therapist.

In women the axillary nodes, located in the armpit, are the primary channels for releasing accumulated lymph from the breasts. Lymphatic breast massage is important and you can do a self breast massage. To learn the technique, you can access an online website <youtube.com/verify_age?next_url=/

watch%3Fv%3Df6jgDk4apog>. I do mine while soaking in an alkaline detox soak.

However, self breast massage may not be right for you if you have radiation burns to the breast or chest area, or if you have had a recent biopsy or lumpectomy. You may have to wait for at least two months for the tissues to heal before massaging the breast for lymphatic drainage.

There's also **dry brush massage** that helps drain the lymphatic system. There's a short demonstration video that will acquaint you with and teach the proper technique for body dry brushing. It really is invigorating. I do mine before I shower or bathe. The YouTube video title is "Dry Skin Brushing Lymphatic System Cleanse Demonstration Video." Please visit this website <youtube.com/watch?v=JoTBP_WJy9E>.

Something to keep in mind is that the brush bristles should be made of *natural plant fibers* and not animal, plastic, or synthetic bristles, which will not give you the desired effects for lymphatic drainage massaging. Also, never get the brush wet; always keep it dry so there can be no mildew or softening of the bristles. Use a separate body brush in the bath or shower.

You must have noticed that I keep referring to *pure* water. Why? Well, municipal drinking water is full of all sorts of chemicals and even toxins, which have negative impact upon our health, immune system, and key organs of elimination, such as the liver, kidneys, plus the spleen to some extent. Yes, the spleen is considered one of the cleansing organs. Please keep in mind that chlorinated solvents, e.g., chlorine and chloramines, in drinking water *act like hormone mimics known as xenoestrogens.*

In my last book, *Our Chemical Lives And The Hijacking Of Our DNA*, available on Amazon.com, I devote an entire chapter, 15, to *Water: Life's Lifeline.* In that chapter I talk about the chemicals that are added to make water potable. Some include chlorine and chloramines, flocculating agents like aluminum-hydroxide, and unsafe fluoride—a protoplasmic poison. Then there are elements that show up in water from pollution like arsenic, barium, heptachlor and heptachlor epoxide, pesticides, etc., and other harmful chemicals.

So, what is *pure* water? It's water that has been filtered as finely as possible. Most pitcher-type water filters don't do very much in filtering. The best and most reliable water filtration process is called *reverse osmosis*, which is installed on the water main where it comes into the house. It's costly but worth it. If you can't afford that, then I suggest obtaining the most effective water purifier device you can afford for the kitchen sink, at least, and use only that water for drinking and cooking your food. There's now available an under-the-kitchen-sink reverse osmosis system available for about $200.00.

Probably one of the most reliable sources for water purifiers that I know about—and have dealt with over the years for non-toxic products—is N.E.E.D.S., which stocks and sells 82 water purifiers in all price ranges. They are out of New York State and you can find them on the Internet at <needs.com/prod_detail_list/eew_Water_Purifiers/a>.

If you get your drinking water from a private well, please make certain that you have your water tested every year—preferably twice a year in these toxic times—for the normal testing parameters plus radioactive particulates, e.g., radon, and especially "fracking chemicals" used in gas extraction from shale deposits.

Under NO circumstances would I recommend drinking distilled (deionized) water. It tends to leach minerals from the body, and should be used only under the guidance of a healthcare practitioner who knows about that aspect of distilled water, which some dispute. However, distilled water is used sometimes in detoxification programs, which must be properly supervised by a well-trained healthcare detox professional.

Water that passes through an entire-household-water-softener, which uses salt as the softening agent, should not be used for drinking or cooking, in my opinion, because of the excess amounts of sodium water passes through that can affect the heart and kidneys.

Water in plastic bottles can contain toxic BPA (Bisphenol-A) used in making plastic, as that chemical tends to leach out of plastic bottles and into the water you drink. To learn more about BPA that also may be in canned foods, I suggest your visiting this website <medicinenet.com/plastic/article.htm>.

Personally, I discourage the use of any plastic materials around food, as food storage containers, and particularly in a microwave oven.

The sun always comes out after a storm.

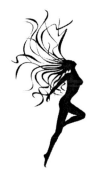

Chapter Twenty-Four
Fatty Acids: Are They Essential?

Cancer patients suffer from a faulty metabolism caused by a mal-function in the lipid defense system. By repairing the lipid defense system the cancer cannot survive. Of course common chemo and radiation causes further harm to the lipid defense system – the very system that protects you from cancer!

…William Kelley Eidem
Author, *The Doctor Who Cures Cancer*

Everyone is exhorted to stay away from fats, which really is misleading, in my opinion. The human body needs healthy fats to be healthy. We can get fats from various sources, most of which are unhealthy and cause health problems. Two fats—*essential fatty acids* (EFAs)—are expressly necessary for health maintenance. They are:

- *Alpha linolenic acid,* an Omega-3 fatty acid, and
- *Linoleic acid,* an Omega-6 fatty acid.

Why are these fats so important in our *daily* diet? Research and published papers reveal they:

- Affect many inflammatory responses and cellular activity.
- Provide cellular signaling.
- Activate and inhibit DNA transcription factors.
- Affect our mood and behavior. Low dietary Omega-3 fatty acids are linked with depression.

Most cooking oils are polyunsaturated or monounsaturated (olive oil). Keep in mind that the optimum healthful ratio of Omega-6 (n-6) to Omega-3 (n-3) should be ***more Omega-3 n-3*** than Omega-6 n-6, or a ratio range of one-to-one to one-to-four (1:1 to 1:4).

Here are the ratios of Omega-6 (n-6) to Omega-3 (n-3) in the more popular cooking and vegetable oils.

Canola: 2 (n-6) to 1 (n-3)

Furthermore, most canola is genetically modified to withstand Glyphosate pesticide, which is sprayed in inordinate amounts on GMO-canola.

Corn: 46 (n-6) to 1 (n-3)

Most corn is *bt*-corn, genetically modified to grow its own herbicide *Bacillus Thuringiensis*.

Cottonseed: just about none to none.

Most cotton crops are genetically modified *bt*-cotton that grows its own herbicide *Bacillus Thuringiensis*.

Olive: 13 (n-6) to 1 (n-3)

Soybean: 7 (n-6) to 1 (n-3)

Most soybeans (87-90% in USA) are genetically modified to withstand Glyphosate pesticide, which is sprayed in inordinate amounts on GMO-soy.

Peanut: almost none to none

Another way of looking at the ratio of Omega-6 to Omega-3, is to consider the percentages of those fatty acids in various oils:

Oil	Omega-6	Omega-3
Canola	20%	9%
Corn	54%	0%
Cottonseed	50%	0%
Soybean	51%	7%
Peanut	32%	0%
Flaxseed oil	14%	57%

If you are taking specific medications like blood thinners or phenothiazine drugs, please check with your physician FIRST about taking fatty acid supplementation.

Never use flaxseed oil as cooking oil. Heat destroys Omega-3 fatty acids.

It's apparent from the above ratios that the average American diet is deficient in Omega-3 EFAs. It seems Americans consume excessive and more quantities of Omega-6 fatty acids than they should for good health. To which I would also add this: Most oils are consumed in the form of burned oils, which are *pro-oxidants* that produce free radicals, from deep-fried foods that generate polycyclic aromatic hydrocarbons (PACs), known carcinogens.

According to the University of Maryland Medical Center,

> *A healthy diet should consist of roughly **2 - 4 times fewer omega-6 fatty acids than omega-3 fatty acids.** The typical American diet, however, tends to contain 14 - 25 times more omega-6 fatty acids than omega-3 fatty acids.* [105] [CJF emphasis added]

However there is one vegetable source, ***flaxseed oil***, which has an excellent ratio of Omega-6 (n-6) to Omega-3 (n-3) EFAs. Make certain the flaxseed is organically grown as some flax has been genetically modified, I understand.

Additionally, flaxseed oil has another specific health benefit, particularly in managing breast cancer and treatment:

Lignans

> *As previously mentioned flaxseed contains lignans. Lignan compounds, which may be found in other seeds and grains, are converted in the body into hormone-like molecules. These molecules have been found to provide some protection against breast cancer. Other benefits for women include: reduced dry eyes, hot flashes, help with ovulation and balancing the hormones.*
>
> *The lignans are recognised [sic] as antioxidants and beneficial for viral, fungal and bacterial infections.* [106]

Furthermore, the percentage of Omega-3 (n-3), *a-linolenic acid* (ALA) in flaxseed is a little over 18 percent, which provides an excellent ratio in the nutritional supplement known as *"high lignan flaxseed oil."* Other than fish oil, flaxseed and walnuts (about 6 percent n-3) are the only plant sources of *higher* quantities of Omega-3 fatty acids. Butternuts, which are not easy to find nor are they popular in the USA, contain a little over 8 percent ALAs.

One caveat I'd like to add is, *"Make certain the flaxseed oil is high lignan, organic, cold pressed, and refrigerate it once opened."* However, I've taken note that the ratios and percentages seem to vary for oils between different information resources.

Here are two publications regarding the role researchers are finding that fatty acids play in breast cancer.

Effects of n-3 PUFAs on breast cancer cells through their incorporation in plasma membrane.

> *PUFAs are important molecules for membrane order and function; they can modify inflammation-inducible cytokines production, eicosanoid production, plasma triacylglycerol synthesis and gene expression*

CONCLUSIONS:

> *Our results indicate that n-3 PUFA feeding might induce modifications of breast cancer membrane structure that increases the degree of fatty acid unsaturation. This paper*

underlines the importance of nutritional factors on health maintenance and on disease prevention. [107]

Mechanisms of omega-3 fatty acid-induced growth inhibition in MDA-MB-231 human breast cancer cells.

The omega-3 fatty acids, eicosapentaenoic acid (EPA) and docosahexaenoic acid (DHA), inhibit the growth of human breast cancer cells in animal models and cell lines, but the mechanism by which this occurs is not well understood. In order to explore possible mechanisms for the modulation of breast cancer cell growth by omega-3 fatty acids, we examined the effects of EPA and DHA on the human breast cancer cell line MDA-MB-231. Omega-3 fatty acids (a combination of EPA and DHA) inhibited the growth of MDA-MB-231 cells by 30-40% ($p<0.05$) in both the presence and absence of linoleic acid, an essential omega-6 fatty acid. When provided individually, DHA was more potent than EPA in inhibiting the growth of MDA-MB-231 cells ($p<0.05$). EPA and DHA treatment decreased tumor cell proliferation ($p<0.05$), as estimated by decreased [methyl-(3)H]-thymidine uptake and expression of proliferation-associated proteins (proliferating cell nuclear antigen, PCNA, and proliferation-related kinase, PRK). [108]

If I may offer a suggestion for a *cold-pressed*, high lignan flax-seed oil, it would be to check out *Bionatures* at <bionatures.

com/01-66-032info.html> for high quality flaxseed oil with an exceptional ratio of Omega-6 (n-6) to Omega-3 (n-3). What I do is swallow my curcumin/turmeric supplements with flaxseed oil, as curcumin needs fat in order to be digestible and bioavailable to body chemistry. Some folks take curcumin with olive oil. However, I figure since I'm taking the flaxseed oil, I might as well not pass up the opportunity to take one less supplement.

A key factor, besides organic, for me with *Bionatures High Lignan Flax Oil* is that it's cold-pressed, meaning the oil was not extruded using chemicals. Flaxseeds were pressed similarly to the way they press olives to make cold-pressed extra virgin olive oil. Again, another reminder of how important it is to keep chemicals out of a body compromised by cancer. But even more important than that, as far as I am concerned, is the ratio of Omega-6 to Omega-3 fatty acids and its lignan content, as per *Bionatures*:

> Omega-6 Linoleic Acid..............1800 mg per Tablespoon
> Omega-3 Alpha Linoleic Acid......6200 mg per Tablespoon
> Omega-9 Oleic Acid.................2040 mg per Tablespoon
> Lignan (SDG*)......................5-23 mg per Tablespoon

*(*Secoisolariciresinol Diglucoside* is a phytoestrogen with estrogen-like activity, potential anti-cancer role in breast and prostate health)

Pace yourself and just enjoy being YOU.

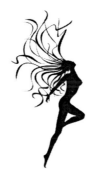

Chapter Twenty-Five
Curcumin, A Spicy Supplement

Oregano is the spice of life.

... Henry J Tillman (1847—1918)
American politician

*P*erhaps that quotation ought to read*, "Curcumin is the spice of life,"* after hearing what it's capable of doing for cancer patients.

More and more conventional scientists are researching the health benefits of holistic supplements, which are naturally occurring components in food that cannot be patented.

However, chemical companies and Big Pharma support genetic modification (GMO) in order to patent foods. Turmeric's curcumin is a food component that neither so far has been genetically modified nor artificially produced. Notwithstanding, the people of India have been using turmeric, the source of curcumin, for ages as part of their delicious and exciting vegetarian cuisine. Turmeric is the yellow colored spice that gives curry powder its rich color and flavor.

In addition to curcumin being successfully investigated in reducing breast cancer cell growth, curcumin has been found to impact certain cellular activity in head and neck cancers. [109]

Curcumin's effectiveness against cancer cells is found in its ability to influence epigenetic modulation, i.e., gene expression at DNA level thereby allowing cancer cells to be killed. [110]

Normal recipe quantities of turmeric cannot supply the amounts needed to impact breast cancer tumor growth. Therapeutic amounts can only be found in nutritional supplementation. For maximum effect, absorption, and bioavailability, which are not well known because of curcumin's inability to be absorbed efficiently by the gut, curcumin supplements should be taken with olive oil to increase its absorption *elevenfold*, according to Dr Russell Blaylock, MD.

Dr Blaylock also recommends emptying the contents of a 500 mg curcumin capsule into a tablespoon of olive oil and mixing it well, then swallowing that mixture. Repeat the procedure AGAIN and take that quantity for *a total of 1,000 mg curcumin in 2 tablespoons olive oil* at least *three times a day* for maximum effect, Dr Blaylock instructed me. According to the instructions I received from Dr Blaylock, he suggests taking curcumin *AFTER* meals and NOT on an empty stomach.

Dr Blaylock also shared with me that his friend's wife was told she had three months to live and no treatment would help her. Are you ready for this? Doctor emailed this to me, *"She has been on a high dose curcumin for the past 15 years and is doing wonderful."* Thank you, Dr Blaylock, for sharing this amazing information with me. I'm listening!

So what are some of the nutritional properties of curcumin? They are numerous and I'm certain that other benefits will be identified with time:

- Helps with the breakdown of toxins in the liver
- Powerful COX-2 anti-inflammatory that can:
  - Stop tumor cell growth
  - Kill tumor cells
  - Prevents growth of new blood vessels
  - Decreases ability of tumors to invade surrounding tissue
  - Turns on tumor *suppression* genes
  - Lowers metastasis risks
- Three hundred times a greater antioxidant than vitamin E
- Stimulates immune system
- Since fat is the main source of the hormone estrogen production post-menopausal, it promotes weight loss
- Reduces estrogenic properties of environmental toxins
- For those taking chemotherapy, it offers protection against its damaging effects
- Works synergistically with green tea. It makes green tea 8 times more effective while green tea makes curcumin's anticancer properties 3 times stronger.
- Turmeric/curcumin is considered the most effective anti-cancer spice

Another spice, saffron with its carotenoid *crocetin*, may be helpful in reducing chemotherapy-induced cellular DNA damage. Research indicates that it has inhibitory effects on the proliferation of certain breast cancer cells: MCF-7 and MDA-MB-231. However, saffron or any of its components *can be toxic* and should *not* be taken in supplement form. It's recommended as a cooking spice only. The Spanish use it in making paella.

Warning: Saffron is not to be taken with any type of blood thinning medications like Coumadin/Warfarin.

Little girls are made of sugar and spice, and every thing nice. Sugar?

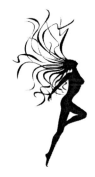

Chapter Twenty-Six
Herbs, Nature's Natural Remedies

For one believeth that he may eat all things: another,
who is weak, eateth herbs.

... Romans 14:2, KJV

Generally speaking, an entire herbal specimen—rather than an isolated compound—is more biologically complex, therefore, there's synergism from all constituent elements within the whole herb rather than in a single isolated element from it, I contend.

A particular organic element may not act as efficaciously without the whole herb companion constituents. That's probably why pharmaceuticals don't work with herbs: they cannot be patented into moneymaking single compound prescription drugs. Botanicals are in the public domain, whereas science-made chemicals and prescription drugs are proprietary assets, usually possessing 'trade secrets', which are patented moneymakers.

Incidentally, herbs have been the human pharmacopoeia since time immemorial. Most of homeopathy is based in botanicals, as are the *Bach Flower Remedies.* Humans have been using herbs since forever. Every culture—even those in antiquity—has recipes handed down from generation to generation, shaman to shaman, medicine woman to medicine woman. How do you think humans were able to get this far in the evolutionary scheme?

If your oncologist or physician is concerned about herb-drug interaction, check out new research indicating that *taking drugs and herbs at different times*—one to two hours apart—may avoid direct interaction within the digestive tract.

Caution: Just like any food product you ingest, allergic reactions can occur *IF* one is allergic to certain substances. Always keep that in mind when ingesting anything, *especially man-made chemicals.* That statement also applies to herbs even though they are natural plants and grown organically.

One possible way to ascertain whether one is allergic to a food is to do what's called 'muscle testing' that some say is non-scientific and others proclaim is 'quackery'. However, in my personal opinion and experience, I feel it is about 98 percent accurate and a probable first line indicator to prevent reactions.

What those who condemn muscle testing don't seem to realize is that the body has *universal knowledge of itself* as a living 'machine' and information 'packets' are relayed along nerve endings and pathways almost instantaneously otherwise, if that were not the case, it probably would take all day to lift a leg.

We are electromagnetic beings and as such, there is much allopathic medicine does not understand about "energy medicine," which, when they do, will become the medicine of the future, I predict.

To do muscle testing as accurately as possible, I feel, place some of the substance being tested under your tongue—similar to nitroglycerin—and then hold your predominant arm perpendicular to your body while another person tries to push the arm down with pressure applied at the wrist area of that extended arm. If the arm cannot be 'broken', i.e., pushed down, that usually means there's no allergic reaction. If the arm 'breaks' (goes down), then there's an almost 100 percent probability that one is allergic to the substance.

However, before performing the muscle test with the substance under the tongue, do a 'dry run' test with nothing in the mouth. The extended arm should be taut and should not 'break'. Then do the muscle test with the substance under the tongue. Both you and the person testing you will experience the difference, if there is a reaction. It's that obvious.

Now, if you want to know how muscle testing feels and works, here's a test you can do on something supposedly benign—table sugar. Do the dry run test first and you should have a firm, unbroken muscle test. Then put a few grains of white table sugar under your tongue and see what happens. Everyone whom I've ever seen tested on table sugar cannot hold the muscle and the arm 'breaks'. Why? Processed white table sugar is nutritionally dangerous to the body, and the body knows it.

If you know you have an allergy to a food, a similar test can be done by placing the food in your unextended, non-dominant hand, clasping it fist-like and placing the fist on the heart area of your body. Then do the muscle test on your extended predominant arm, and see what you get. Believe me, you will know if the test was psychosomatically affected or not because you will know that you could not resist the pressure no matter how hard you tried. The body knows! One thing to remember is this: After a test that 'breaks', remove the item from your mouth or hand, and do a test with nothing and you should get back to normal—no break. Always leave the body with a normal, non-breaking test. Voodoo? No, just inherent body knowledge, and an aspect of energy medicine for which high diagnostic fees cannot be billed to health insurance companies.

Chinese Traditional Medicine Herbs

Chinese Traditional Medicine (CTM) has been practiced and used for close to 5,000 years. Pharmaceutical companies were founded in the late nineteenth and early twentieth centuries—just over a hundred or so years ago.

CTM has been proven to be helpful as an adjuvant treatment with conventional chemotherapy treatment for breast cancer.

The following are traditional CTM herbs for breast cancer management:

Oldenlandia (*Bai Hua She She Cao* in Chinese) is used to treat snakebites, removes toxins and clears the blood, is non-toxic and relieves pain. Encourages cell apoptosis.

Taraxacum, (*pugongying*) is the common dandelion, known for its liver and blood detoxifying properties. Dandelion's *Luteolin* reduces free radicals.

Scutellaria (*banzhi*), a mint family herb known for its toxin removing capabilities and anti-cancer properties.

Aurantium (*Zhi Shi*) bitter orange (Seville orange) acts as a stimulant and may interact unfavorably with prescription statins similar to the way grapefruit acts with some prescription drugs.

Curcuma (*Yu-Jin*) turmeric has anti-tumor properties and relieves edema that many breast surgery patients suffer with post-surgery.

Coix lachryma-jobi or Jobs's tears (*yang-yi-mi*) a relative to maize/corn from which ***Kanglaite*** is made that has been tested in hospitals in China. Results on over 270,000 cancer patients indicate its effectiveness and anti-tumor action against malignant tumors in the breast, liver, lungs, and stomach. It inhibits new tumor cell growth.

Astragalus (*Huang-Qi*) and **Angelica** (*Dang Gui*) both activate the immune system and have anti-tumor properties.

Antineoplastic-like Action Herbs

The following herbs have antineoplastic-like action, which means they are capable of checking the maturation or production of malignant cells, something known to herbalists and shamans—but not by that terminology—before pharmaceutical makers with chemotherapy came on the scene. Nature has been providing therapeutic medicinal plants and herbs since forever.

Chinese Name: ***Bai He She She Cao*** increases phagocytosis by the lymphatics

Common Name: Oldenlandia

Chinese Name: ***Da Huang*** inhibits breast tumor and melanoma cells

Common Name: Rhubarb Root and Rhizome

Chinese Name: ***E Zhu*** cervical cancer

Common Name: Zedoania

Chinese Name: ***Shan Dou Gen*** inhibits malignant cells respiration and toxin removal

Common Name: Sophora Root

Chinese Name: ***Shi Shang Bai*** tumor inhibition

Common Name: Selaginaella

Common Name: **Cleavers** lymphatic drainage

Latin: *Galium aparine*

Common Name: **Mistletoe** antineoplastic activity

Latin: *Viscum alba*

Common Name: **Red Clover** preventative: breast and prostate tumors/cancers

Latin: *Flos Trifolium pratense*

Common Name: ***Pau D'Arco, Lapacho, Taheebo*** anti-cancer and anti-tumor properties

Latin: *Tabebuia impestiginosa*

Common Name: **Sweet Violet** cancer of the skin in particular

Latin: *Flos Viola odorata*

Helpful Herb Hints

Red Clover

This sweet smelling wild flower is dried and usually used to make an herbal tea that is rich in isoflavones, related to flavonoids, and phytoestrogens, those water-soluble elements that act like estrogens in the human body due to being able to fit in as estrogen receptors. This herb also comes in capsules, tablets, and liquid forms.

Red clover is rich in antioxidants, helps to purify the blood, and has a detoxifying effect on the liver and kidneys. However, red clover can interfere with some medications, so be aware of that and discuss it with your oncologist or holistic physician first.

Milk Thistle

The efficacy of herbs cannot be disputed even though Big Pharma, who makes chemical pharmaceuticals, often disputes herbal potencies and potentialities. An excellent case in point is the herb Milk Thistle substance *silibinin* that was efficacious in treating four people suffering with wild amanita mushroom poisoning in the Washington, DC area in September 2011. They were treated at Georgetown University Medical Center. Silibinin, flavonolignans from silymarin in Milk Thistle, prevented liver damage. To appreciate this remarkable natural pharmacological discussion, visit online <foodsafetynews.com/2011/10/milk-thistle-extract-combats-mushroom-poisoning/?utm_source=newsletter&utm_medium=email&utm_campaign=111010>.

Milk Thistle *may be* helpful to reduce liver involvement and detoxification from chemotherapy. Always check with your healthcare provider before taking any herb while taking chemotherapy, as there can be some contraindications with some chemo drugs.

Milk Thistle is one herb that can induce an allergic reaction in some people. Other herbs that can cause allergic reaction are dandelion, stinging nettle, and burdock.

Essiac Herbal Formula

This is a specialized formula of burdock root, sheep sorrel leaves, slippery elm bark, and Indian rhubarb root that a Canadian nurse formulated many years ago and which cancer patients find extremely helpful in supporting the immune system.

The product comes as a finely ground dehydrated powder herbal that has to be prepared in a special manner. It comes from Canada and I've been using it almost from day one of my odyssey. There are fake and knockoff Essiac Teas, so one has to be careful to get the real deal from Essiac Canada International, Inc., P.O. Box 23155, Ottawa, Ont., Canada, K2A 4E2 Email: info@essiaccanada.ca.

Herbal Detox Tea

Traditional Medicinals® puts out an herbal tea that "promotes healthy liver function"—Lemon Every Day Detox® containing the following organic herbs: burdock root, stinging nettle leaf, cleavers, dandelion, and lemon myrtle leaf, which I found wonderful for my protocol. It's caffeine-free and comes in individual tea bags.

Herbal Science

Herbs have been on the face of the earth probably before humans came along. Herbs go back in time, history, and the archives of numerous civilizations and cultures. Aromatic and healing plants have been used as medicine as far back as humans can remember.

The Bible mentions herbs. The Egyptians used them. Ayurvedic medicine has been using herbs for thousands of years. Shamans and medicine men and women have employed them. Herbs have become part of the human healing legacy.

Knowledge about their healing powers has been handed down from generation to generation even without efficacy studies having been done because they were proven over millennia to be efficacious in healing the human body. Those facts were recognized and catalogued into herbal pharmacopoeias. Here is a listing of some of those pharmacopoeias:

Austrian Pharmacopoeia
British Herbal Pharmacopoeia
British Pharmacopoeia
European Pharmacopoeia
French Pharmacopoeia
German Drug Codex
German Pharmacopoeia
Indian Herbal Pharmacopoeia
Japanese Pharmacopoeia
Pharmacopoeia of the People's Republic of China
United States Pharmacopeia
United States Pharmacopeia National Formulary

Herbs Used As Bath Soaks

Several herbs can be used in bath water as a soaking agent. *Lavender* not only is pungently pleasing, it induces relaxation. This type of a soak just may be what "the doctor orders" to get relaxed before bedtime and to be able to forego a sleeping pill.

Other relaxing soaking herbs include **chamomile** and non-sprayed **rose petals**. Some herbs like the mint family and rosemary can be stimulating—something you may not want before bedtime.

Detoxifying Soaks

Herbal

There are detoxifying soaks. One herb that can be used for that purpose is **Pau d'Arco,** the South American herb. *Pau d'Arco* also can be used as an anti-fungal foot soak.

Alkaline Soak

There's a caveat that comes with the following information, and it is this: Make certain you have discussed this soak with your holistic health practitioner and that your body can handle it, since it requires soaking for at least 20 minutes in very warm water with **Epsom salts and baking soda,** which your heart must be in condition to handle, I feel. You may feel weak after the soak, so be forewarned.

The soak that I used was one-quarter (1/4) cup Epsom salts and one-quarter (1/4) cup baking soda dissolved in a tub of as warm water as I could tolerate. Sink down into the tub and allow the water to come up to your chin for 20 minutes. You may have to add some hot water at the 10-minute mark.

After 20 minutes, drain the tub and rinse off your body with warm water. Dry yourself, put on pajamas and immediately crawl into bed under heavy covers to sweat off toxins. In the beginning it will feel as though nothing is happening. About ten minutes in bed, sweat ought to start pouring out of you. Stay under the covers for at least 30 minutes relaxing and detoxifying.

Warning

It is my recommendation that the alkaline detoxifying soak should not be done more than twice a week and at least 3 days apart. Furthermore, patients with diabetes, hypertension (high blood pressure), and balance problems must check with their managing physician before embarking on the alkaline soak ritual. Patients taking chemotherapy many not want to do this soak, as it can remove the chemo. However, if you have given up on chemo and want to detox it, then this soak may be for you. Talk with your holistic physician before doing it.

Herbs, I wouldn't know what to do without them.

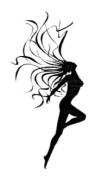

Chapter Twenty Seven
Sea Vegetables and Fucoidan

Love is like seaweed; even if you have pushed it away,
you will not prevent it from coming back.

… Nigerian Proverb

*M*ost westerners are not familiar with edible sea vegetables—seaweed—as a food item. Asian cultures, especially the Japanese, have relied on these wonderful gifts from the sea for ages to supply nutrients, particularly what is referred to as trace minerals. Seaweed sometimes is called algae. Would you believe that seaweed is used as food, fertilizer, and medicine? Seaweed is valued particularly for its rich source of naturally occurring iodine needed for thyroid function and to prevent goiter.

Regarding seaweed being used as food, records going back to 300 BCE indicate it was used as food in ancient China. Needless to say, most coastal cultures have been harvesting sea vegetables ever since they can remember. Numerous cultures harvest seaweed and some apply it as fertilizer to their growing fields to enrich the soil. *Wikipedia* even shows a photograph of seaweed used to thatch a roof on a house in Denmark.

The importance of seaweed in our diet—and the breast cancer patient's diet in particular—is understated, I feel, especially since most western eating 'styles' are saturated with processed foods that lack trace minerals, which seaweed has in abundance, and are needed for good health.

The macrobiotic diet for the management of cancer includes seaweed, especially *Kombu.* However, there are numerous varieties of seaweed, a few of which I list below. You may be familiar with a couple, especially if you like Japanese food, as I do. One of my favorite Japanese dishes—also that of my late husband—is miso soup with loads of *Miyok (Undaria pinnatifida)* seaweed floating in it, eaten with steamed brown rice, *Agedashi Dofu,* and seaweed salad. Oh such yummy comfort food—for me, that was—when we would go out to eat, which was not that often.

Since most seaweed comes dried, it has to be soaked in water at least 5 to 10 minutes before using it in a recipe, or add it dry and diced while cooking soup.

Arame: sweet, mild taste, delicious alone or sautéed with land vegetables

Dulse: use as a condiment instead of salt. Sprinkle on soups, salads, and veggies

Hijiki: one of the most mineral rich of all sea vegetables
See my recipe for *Hijiki Salad* in Chapter 20.

Kelp: used in powder form as a salt substitute or condiment

Kombu: use for slow cooking soups, beans, and stews. It tenderizes, adds flavor, and makes beans easier to digest with no flatulence after eating.*Kombu* also can be used to make a quick stock: To 4 cups of water add 1 strip *Kombu,* bring to a boil and simmer 4 minutes. Remove *Kombu,* which may be bitter tasting after simmering, and use the flavorful stock.

Nori: usually pressed into dried sheets that Japanese chefs use to create hand rolls (*Temaki*), *Gunkan* (small rice cups with fish egg topping usually), *Norimaki* (numerous varieties of sushi rolls).

Wakame: the seaweed most often added to miso soup.

There's something I'd like to caution you about regarding seaweed recipes: *most use vinegar, particularly rice vinegar,* which I definitely do NOT recommend on the cancer elimination diet, as vinegar turns body pH to acid and 'excites' candida or yeast growth, something we want to eliminate and keep under total control.

Fucoidan: some exciting information about seaweed and cancer.

Seaweed comes in many colors, shapes, and sizes. In *brown* seaweed the polysaccharide *fucoidan*—rich in calcium, iodine, iron, selenium, zinc to name a few—has been found to improve the immune system and, more importantly according to research, causes cancer cells to self-destruct or what medically is termed apoptosis or 'cell suicide'—how about '*hari kari*', the ancient form of suicide defeated samurai would employ to restore their honor, since I've discussing some things Japanese. The actual Japanese term, though, is "*hara kiri.*"

That's not the only excitement surrounding *fucoidan.* It's capable of enhancing natural killer (NK) cells activity within the body, which go after cancer cells and kill 'em dead. The upside is that *fucoidan* does not damage healthy cells, as chemotherapy often does, and you can take *fucoidan* in supplement form, which I do.

Other ancillary ingredients in brown seaweed also are thought to have the ability to burn off visceral fat—between abdominal organs, which I refer to as 'fat bumpers'—a most likely site where toxins store and also can be difficult to detoxify since we can't 'exercise' fat bumpers per se. Thermogenesis would be the metabolic process involved that speeds up the metabolic rate to burn off visceral fat. *Fucoidan,* I think, also helps in the detoxification process because of a probable ability to help detoxify visceral fat.

Japanese warriors going into battle would shout, *"Banzai."* Maybe each time we sit down to eat some seaweed or take a *fucoidan* supplement we ought to say to ourselves, *"Banzai,"* as we fight the good fight to overcome breast cancer cells.

Life is a bowl of cherries; just don't concentrate on the pits.

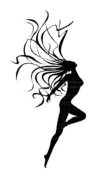

Chapter Twenty-Eight
Vitamin D and Breast Cancer

*This is like the Holy Grail of cancer medicine;
vitamin D produced a drop in cancer rates greater
than that for quitting smoking, or indeed
any other countermeasure in existence.*

**… Dennis Mangan
Clinical laboratory scientist**

This chapter will be easy for me to write since I'm just going with the science on Vitamin D and not many opinions since I differ with the emerging science. I consider some of the daily and weekly values recommended to be in extreme ranges and here's my rationale for that:

As Nature intends, vitamin D is manufactured mostly during the bio-chemical reaction of sunlight with cholesterol under the skin. Ten minutes of noontime sun-rays on a fair skinned person produces about 10,000 international units of vitamin D. Staying in the sun for long periods produces sunburn, which is Nature's way of telling us we are getting too much vitamin D and cool it. Make sense?

It is my opinion, however, that taking mega doses of vitamin D at one time overloads the liver and *may* cause some toxicity since vitamin D is fat soluble. There are five forms of vitamin D:

Vitamin D$_1$ Ergocalciferol with lumisterol
Vitamin D$_2$ Ergocalciferol made from ergosterol
Vitamin D$_3$ Cholecalciferol made from dehydrocholesterol under the skin
Vitamin D$_4$ 22-dihydroergocalciferol
Vitamin D$_5$ Sitocalciferol made from irradiated 7-dehydrositosterol

According to *Wikipedia,*

> *Vitamin D$_2$ is a derivative of ergosterol, a membrane sterol named for the ergot fungus, which is produced by some organisms of phytoplankton, invertebrates, and fungi. The vitamin ergocalciferol (D$_2$) is produced in these organisms from ergosterol in response to UV irradiation. D$_2$ is not produced by land plants or vertebrates, because they lack the precursor ergosterol. The biological fate for producing 25(OH)D from vitamin D$_2$ is expected to be the same as for D$_3$, although some controversy exists over whether or not D$_2$ can fully substitute for vitamin D$_3$ in the human diet.* [111]

Fish oil—cod liver oil, in particular, for ages—is an excellent source of vitamin D since fish metabolize sunlight in the plankton, krill, etc. they eat as food sources. Basically it comes down to 'ingesting and converting light molecules'. Plants do something similar with sunlight rays through the process of photosynthesis. So why is it that everyone seems paranoid about sunlight and does everything to block it, especially those chemtrails sprayed in the sky and the fixation with sunscreens that don't allow sun rays to penetrate and make vitamin D, but, what in effect they obviously do, is drive toxic sunscreen chemicals into the skin from the sun's heat rays interaction with open pores on the skin—at least that's my opinion.

Some people who take vitamin D mega doses *may* lose their hair, which indicates a toxicity of sorts building up, as far as I'm concerned. I happen to know that from personal experience. I can't take heavy-duty doses of vitamin D. Some other symptoms of vitamin D overload are nausea, vomiting, loss of appetite, high blood pressure, kidney malfunction, and an overall failure to thrive, which is catastrophic for anyone with any form of cancer. However, we DO need sufficient vitamin D for good health.

My major concern for my readers is that if you are taking vitamin D—and I think 20 minutes of sunshine a day and a diet high in vitamin D foods, which cannot form a toxic reaction, or a natural supplement like cod liver oil capsules—just may be sufficient *unless* a specific blood test for vitamin D levels shows deficiency. All holistic physicians respect the need for vitamin D levels and that would be one of the very first blood draws they would prescribe.

I heartily recommend you make certain the vitamin D you are taking comes from the most natural sources possible, e.g., fish oil, some vegetables, free-range eggs, and sunshine. Steering away from synthetic forms of vitamin D, in my opinion, should be a no-brainer. Most processed foods include synthetic vitamin D. Perhaps you may appreciate knowing that synthetic vitamin D in processed foods probably can't be assimilated properly because many of the co-factors and enzymes needed for biosynthesis may be missing.

Another aspect of vitamin D or any vitamin, mineral, enzyme, co-enzyme, etc. in food crops and plants is the role that genetic modification—GM—plays. I don't think anyone really knows the impact upon a plant's ability to produce vitamin D or other nutrients as a result of its seed genes having been genetically modified either through Transgenic or Cisgenic gene transfer. That alone could be a factor in less nutrient rich foods and diets. That's why I'm a proponent of organic and sustainable agriculture and animal husbandry, plus the labeling of GMO ingredients on food labels.

In my opinion as a retired *natural* nutritionist that's a problem with processed foods: Most naturally occurring nutrients are processed out. White flour is an excellent example. Usually it is 'fortified' with synthetically produced vitamins that the body cannot 'recognize' and metabolize thereby creating deficiencies and disease-inducing conditions and/or overloading the liver and kidneys with toxins.

A classic example is vitamin C's molecular structure $C_3H_4O_3$ compared with ascorbic acid, synthetic vitamin C, whose molecular structure is $C_6H_8O_6$. Both vitamin C molecular structures demonstrate what in chemistry is called "mirror images" or *chirality*. *"Nature requires that all chemicals be receptive; bond to each other; interact; get assimilated and/or transmuted into other biochemicals or reagents. In turn, those inter-reactions propel or synthesize molecular and cellular life. Those processes should not cause cellular damage. That's the way it's always been,"* as I said in my last book, *Our Chemical Lives And The Hijacking Of Our DNA.*

However, it ought to be noted that of the various stereoisometric forms of ascorbic acid (synthetic vitamin C), only one form identical to natural vitamin C produces the same anti-ascorbutic results or activity, even though the other forms have strong anti-oxidant properties.

Now, compare the molecular structures for *natural* vitamin C and *synthetic* vitamin C, ascorbic acid.

The Science About Vitamin D

In *Our Chemical Lives And The Hijacking Of Our DNA, A Probe Into What's Probably Making Us Sick,* I discuss the impact of man-made chemicals on our chromosome's telomeres, which are at both ends of each chromosome, that when damaged, is where cancer cells often take root. Telomeres protect each chromosome from being compromised by whatever, and the longer in length they remain, the more healthy and safe a chromosome is. Keeping in mind that telomeres get shorter or 'get lost' as cells divide, there is an enzyme, *telomerase,* responsible for reconstructing telomeres. When that reconstruction doesn't happen efficiently or there is a deficiency in telomerase, disease patterns can strike and/or the aging process becomes prominent.

In October 2011 scientists at the Georgia Health Sciences University revealed that vitamin D could increase telomerase activity by 19 percent. Furthermore, the study's scientists said, "*Our data suggest that vitamin D may improve telomere maintenance and prevent cell senescence.*" Since vitamin D is a major tool in Mother Nature's tool kit for health, maintenance, and repair of the human body, it's comforting to know that science and technology are beginning to catch up with Mother Nature. Soon science will find that similar mechanisms are at work with all nutrients in naturally grown food. That's why Creator God and Nature put them there and not petro-chemicals, pharmaceuticals, or vaccines. You can't fool Mother Nature!

One vitamin D paper that you may want to know about is "Vitamin D and breast cancer: interpreting current evidence" by Rowan T Chlebowski of the Los Angeles Biomedical Research Institute in Torrance, California. That paper was published in *Breast Cancer Research* 2011, 13:217. You may read that paper online at <breast-cancere-research.com/content/13/4/217>. It's quite lengthy but here's the last paragraph from the *Conclusion* section:

Current evidence is sufficient to support further study of factors influencing 25(OH)D levels, associations between 25(OH)D levels and breast cancer in premenopausal and Black women, moderate dose (≤2,000 IU D$_3$/day) supplemental vitamin D use and breast cancer incidence, and observational studies evaluating whether a threshold higher 25(OH)D level is associated with adverse clinical outcome in women with breast cancer. Before routine clinical application of any strategies targeting vitamin D status for breast cancer prevention or therapy are undertaken, the limitations of the current evidence should be considered.

To understand more about the importance of vitamin D in health, you may want to read the article "41 International Scientists & Physicians Call For New Recommendations for Vitamin D" at <healthmaven.blogspot.com/2010/07/vitamin-d-is-essential-for-prevention.html>.

The author of this book, in her opinion, agrees wholeheartedly, and suggests you discuss vitamin D supplementation with your physician—you need it, but what's the right amount for you? That can only be determined by a blood test, I think. Furthermore, some news about vitamin D was breaking while I was writing this book. It concerns too much vitamin D that can and may cause the heart to beat too fast and out of rhythm—atrial fibrillation. Please see the warning about too much vitamin D and what it can do to your heart at this online site <msnbc.msn.com/id/45325473/ns/health-diet_and_nutrition/t/

vitamin-d-warning-too-much-can-harm-your-heart/from/
toolbar?#.TsRxlz25PRk>.

*God made the sun to shine for everyone, so enjoy it
every day.*

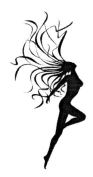

Vitamins, Minerals, and Amino Acids: Their Roles in Cancer Management

The chemicals that are running our body and our brain are the same chemicals that are involved in emotion. And that says to me that . . . we'd better pay more attention to emotions with respect to health.

… Candace Pert, PhD (1946—)
American neuroscientist & pharmacologist

The Mineral Selenium

There's quite a bit of information about the toxicity of selenium, a trace mineral necessary for a healthy body and, in particular, to thwart cancer cells from forming as a result of free radical production. Free radical production is a naturally occurring process in the human body, particularly in digestion and assimilation of the foods, countering chemicals, additives, sugar, and other things we force our bodies to use as 'nutrition'. Selenium's superior capability to battle cancer cells and ward off cancer is because of the *essential component of glutathione peroxidase,* the enzyme required for the body to produce glutathione, one of the most powerful antioxidants known to date.

In my last book, *Our Chemical Lives And The Hijacking Of Our DNA,* when discussing selenium I said, *"The mineral selenium demonstrates if a little bit is good; a lot more is bad. This trickster has been promoted as a panacea at times; whereas, it should be regarded with much respect. Most folks fall into the category of over supplementing with the nutritional supplement.*

"...One of the adverse side effects of selenium toxicity (selenosis) is severe hair loss. ...Many electronic items "burn off" selenium when they heat up. ...If you are taking a special selenium dietary supplement without a health care professionals advice and supervision, STOP immediately, please, and obtain reliable information about what to do so that you can prevent problems with your health."

Selenoproteins in food have antioxidant properties that prevent free radical damage. In my opinion, the best—and safest—source of selenium is dietary from organically grown food sources such as Brazil nuts that can have as much as 544 mcg of selenium in one *ounce* of raw Brazil nuts. One medium size organic egg can have 14 mcg. The Recommended Daily Allowances (RDAs) for males and females over 19 years of age is 55 mcg a day. During pregnancy, the RDAs are 60 mcg/day, while during lactation, 70 mcg/day.

Selenomethionine (*organic* selenium analogue of the amino acid methionine) found in foods, particulary high selenium yeasts, is the safest form of selenium to take, I think. But keep in mind it is YEAST, something breast cancer patients want to steer clear of, in my opinion. However, body chemistry can utilize selenomethionine more efficiently because of its protein/amino acid analogue.

According to the Office of Dietary Supplements, National Institutes of Health,

> *This form of selenium was used in the large scale cancer prevention trial in 1983, which demonstrated that taking a daily supplement containing 200 micrograms of selenium per day could lower the risk of developing prostate, lung, and colorectal cancer.* *

However, during my management protocol for breast cancer, I have been eating as many as five organically grown Brazil nuts a day that started at the twelfth week of my program. I would eat them after having had a meal for better incorporation within the bolus of food being processed in the stomach. Since I was on a six-week detox program, I had

---

* Clark LC, Combs Jr GF, Turnbull BW, Slate EH, Chalker D, Chow J, Davis LS, Glover RA, Graham GF, Gross EG, Krongrad A, Lesher JL, Park HK, Sanders BB, Smith CL, Taylor JR. Effects of selenium supplementation for cancer prevention in patients with carcinoma of the skin. A randomized controlled trial. J Am Med Assoc 1996;276:1957-63.

elected not to do anything with selenium until I had finished detoxifying.

Safety Issues Surrounding Nutritional Supplements

In February 2011 I wrote an article for *VacTruth.com* titled "Vaccines Can't Claim What Nutritional Supplements Can: No Deaths!" that you can read at <vactruth.com/2011/02/22/vaccines-can%e2%80%99t-claim-what-nutritional-supplements-can-no-deaths/>.

The interesting spin that nutritional supplements cause health problems is taken out of context, in my opinion, because *any* substance when abused or not used correctly can cause harm. Examples: Air, we can't live without it, but when air bubbles get into a vein, we may not live. The body needs water to live, but water in the lungs will kill. It's all a matter of proper context and use, and nutritional supplementation is no different, particularly for those who don't want to understand nutrient physiology or, perhaps, believe that man-made chemicals are best for the body because Big Pharma makes, sells and does the 'science' on them, plus provides generous commissions for MDs writing prescriptions.

The *Orthomolecular Medicine News Service* sent out a press release January 5, 2011 that emphasized the statistical facts regarding supplement safety.

Zero Deaths from Vitamins, Minerals, Amino Acids or Herbs

Poison Control Statistics Prove Supplements' Safety Yet Again (OMNS Jan 5, 2011) There was not even one death caused by a dietary supplement in 2009, according to the most recent information collected by the U.S. National Poison Data System.

The new 200-page annual report of the American Association of Poison Control Centers, published in the journal Clinical Toxicology, shows zero deaths from multiple vitamins; zero deaths from any of the B vitamins; zero deaths from vitamins A, C, D, or E; and zero deaths from any other vitamin.

Additionally, there were no deaths whatsoever from any amino acid, herb, or dietary mineral supplement.

Two people died from non-nutritional mineral poisoning, one from a sodium salt and one from an iron salt or iron. On page 1139, the AAPCC report specifically indicates that the iron fatality was not from a nutritional supplement. One other person is alleged to have died from an "Unknown Dietary Supplement or Homeopathic Agent." This claim remains speculative, as no verification information was provided.

60 poison centers provide coast-to-coast data for the U.S. National Poison Data System, "one of the few real-time national surveillance systems in existence, providing a model public health surveillance system for all types of exposures, public health event identification, resilience response and situational awareness tracking."

Over half of the U.S. population takes daily nutritional supplements. Even if each of those people took only one single tablet daily, that makes 155,000,000 individual doses per day, for a total of nearly 57 billion doses annually. Since many persons take more than just one vitamin or mineral tablet, actual consumption is considerably higher, and the safety of nutritional supplements is all the more remarkable.

---

*If nutritional supplements are allegedly so "dangerous," as the FDA and news media so often claim, then **where are the bodies?*** [CJF emphasis added]

However, in contrast we find that deaths from prescription drug overdose in Florida between the years 2003-2009 were discussed in a *Journal of the American Medical Association (JAMA).* [112] Non-suicidal deaths from prescription drug overdose increased 325 percent during those six years. Interesting? So what's the problem about nutritional supplements?

To be fair and equitable in my reporting, I must include that there have been relatively few adverse event reports (AERs) described relative to nutritional supplements, which the Alliance for Natural Health reported:

Furthermore, the number of supplement AERs is quite low—only 1,080 in 2008. And keep in mind that over half the US population (at least 154 million individuals) take nutritional supplements, according to data from 2007 National Health Interview Survey. The supplement AER figure is even lower when compared to the 526,527 prescription drug AERs in 2008. In other words, for every adverse event from supplements, there are 488 adverse events from prescription drugs! [113]

Did you note the number of adverse event reports for prescription drugs in 2008: 526,527—that's over half a million. So what does that say about the safety of prescription drugs versus the safety of nutritional supplements?

The Vitamin Doctor
The Opinions of David Juan, MD

To be both objective and in some ways subjective regarding nutritional supplementation, please allow me to introduce Dr David Juan's video because he makes a valid point, and something I have been a proponent of since studying *natural nutrition,* which is nutrient interaction, especially during this, the 'chemical age' in which we live.

You may access his video online at <doctorshealthpress. com/video/vd/?sb=FREEDOM&date=12012011>.

Historically, culturally, and agriculturally, nutrients have been an intrinsic part of the food chain, which ancient cultures recognized and used either as herbs or special foods in specific quantities as supplements for healing and the maintenance of overall good health.

However, before the Industrial Revolution there were no other interfering biochemical factors, e.g., food processing, 'enrichment supplements', fluoridated and chemicalized drinking water, pharmaceutical drugs and vaccines, chemotherapy, and ubiquitous pollution from every aspect of science and technology (chemtrails) that impact the human immune system, which, in turn, requires a reassessment of how nutrients interact. Dr Juan seems to have done more of that type of assessment and provides some of his findings in "Foods You Should Never Mix With Popular Supplements" in his video.

The first nutrient discussed is selenium and selenosis, which I talked about earlier in this chapter. Iron is next.

I truly believe too many processed foods are 'enriched' with it. The late Carl C Pfeiffer, MD, PhD (1908–1988), a medical doctor and biochemist who researched schizophrenia, allergies, and other diseases, also thought that food processing iron enrichment should have been discontinued. Too much iron contributes to *hemachromatosis,* which damages the liver. Personally, I think too much iron also could be part of the celiac syndrome that causes severe abdominal problems from eating gluten. Interestingly, when gluten—abundant in wheat flour that is 'enriched'—is taken out of the diet, those awful symptoms subside. Perhaps it's the intake of non-bioavailable iron that also could have been contributing to the syndrome's symptoms. Ever think of that?

In Chapter 28 I discussed my thoughts and concerns regarding vitamin D. Dr Juan's video may help my readers understand the *bioavailability* differences between *real foods extract* vitamin/mineral nutrients/supplements and *synthetic/chemical* supplements, which are not 100 percent bioavailable and can cause the liver to be overtaxed.

The paramount importance of nutrient-rich, organically grown foods in the diet ought to become obvious as *the key* in managing and healing breast cancer, or any cancer for that matter.

Amino Acids

Back in the early 1980s I wrote the book *Understanding Body Chemistry and Hair Mineral Analysis* wherein I discussed my thoughts on the future of medicine and that it just may lie in amino acids, those compounds that 'direct' body functions from a neuro-chemical aspect that originates within the human brain. Dr Candace Pert, PhD, is one of the pioneers who worked in that field of research, and her work has produced much to think about, particularly in the field of neuroscience.

However, numerous other researchers, academicians, and medical doctors also have found amino acids efficacious in the treatment of disease, and cancer in particular. One such medical doctor is Stanislaw Burzynski, MD, PhD, who uses antineoplastons, which are peptide and amino acid derivatives that he discovered and do work in curing cancers.

Other physicians may employ amino acids in the treatment of cancer, including breast, along with the treatment and management of serious and chronic diseases such as Addison's disease, Glommerulonephritis, Multiple Sclerosis, Myasthenia Gravis (Lou Gerhig's disease), Rheumatoid Arthritis, and a host of autoimmune disorders.

Patients need to keep in mind that amino acid treatment/therapy probably cannot be employed while taking corticosteroid drugs such as Prednisone, which tend to suppress the immune system, or while on a regimen of cancer chemotherapeutic drugs, e.g., Cyclosporin or Methotrexate. Amino acid therapy builds up or enhances the immune system, so there could be a biochemistry conflict as a result of taking both simultaneously, or at least that's my opinion.

Amino acids and peptides (small size proteins)—because of their innate importance in body chemistry—can be considered as the building blocks of life. They also may be considered as "immunomodulators," keys for enhancing the immune system to attack and fight cancer cell production and/or promote *apoptosis*, a cell process whereby cells play an active part in their own deaths, e.g., 'cell suicide'. Amino acids are body and patient friendly, since human bodies have been producing them for eons.

Don't rock the boat if you don't know how to swim.

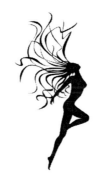

Chapter Thirty
Clothing and Cancer: Is There A Connection?

Be careless in your dress if you will, but keep a tidy soul.

… **Mark Twain (1835—1910)**
American humorist & author

N o doubt you've heard the aphorism, "Dressed to kill."
Well, there may be more to that than meets the eye,
as they say. How come? First off, new clothing for the last two
or three decades has been impregnated with sizing or finishing chemicals that are toxic, some of which include bromines,
caustic soda, formaldehyde, halogens, sulfonamides, sulfuric
acid, and urea resins.

Furthermore, clothing imported from cheap labor manufacturing countries often contains long-lasting disinfectants
that are extremely difficult to remove—even with several launderings. Some have distinctive odors similar to bug spray or
diesel. Almost all new clothing has a perfume-like odor [toxic
chemicals] that should be removed before wearing, as it causes

immunologic stress either from breathing the out gassing fumes or from contact with the skin.

Some clothing even may contain flame retardant chemicals, which are known to cause neurological damage in rat studies. Even though Brominated Tris, a mutagen that causes cancer and sterility in animals, was banned from children's clothing in 1977, it still can be found in upholstered furniture foam, baby carriers, and bassinets. Newer flame-retardants survive as many as 50 launderings. PBDEs have been shown in studies to cause brain damage, ADHD symptoms, and fertility problems.

Never place flame retardant clothing on a baby nor place a baby into a crib with flame retardant bedding, in my opinion, as they must breathe in the toxins and rub their skin and fingers on the fabric and then put them into their little mouths. LL Bean and Land's End, as far as I can gather, sell children's sleepwear without flame-retardants. There is a natural 'flame retardant' type fabric—wool, from which crib padding and mattress covers are made. Online purveyors like Dream SoftBedware.com sell numerous bed and bath linens, comforters, organic wool bedding, and so much more. If you want more information about them, you may visit DreamSoftBedware.com online at <dreamsoftbedware.com/coyuchi.html?clid=CI30hv6D8awCFUXf4Aod-ROyfA>.

Here's a field guide to what most likely is in finishing or sizing chemicals:

- Acrylic, wrinkle free, easy care, polyester, and shrinkage free garments: formaldehyde

- Water repellent: fluoropolymers as in Teflon
- Moth-proof or mildew resistant: Bacterial and fungicidal chemicals, formaldehyde
- Civilian outdoor wear and military uniforms: the insecticide permethrin
- Polyester, acrylic, and nylon fabrics are close cousins to plastic
- Spandex, or elastane, is a synthetic fiber (polyurethane-polyurea copolymer) known for its elasticity
- Rayon, which is made from wood cellulose steeped in caustic soda (sodium hydroxide) and acid baths, is not environmentally friendly especially during the viscose manufacture process, as a lot of water and air are polluted.

Breast cancer patients, please take note that there have been lawsuits filed alleging high levels of formaldehyde in *Victoria's Secret* bras. For more information about that, you may want to visit <yourlawyer.com/topics/overview/Victorias_Secret_Bra_Rash> and read "Victoria's Secret Bra Defect Injury Lawsuits" that talks about rash, hives, chemicals, and formaldehyde in bras.

Whether you know it or not, dyes and chemicals in fabrics can be absorbed through the skin. Toxic out gas fumes constantly are breathed into the body thereby causing tissue damage to sinuses, bronchi, and lungs in addition to burdening the body with toxic chemicals—something a breast cancer patient does not need to complicate matters.

Then there's the issue of laundry detergent residues that are left in laundered clothing. One laundry detergent constituent, sodium tripolyphosphate, *may* be absorbed through contact with the skin. No studies have confirmed that, but it's better to be forewarned about a possibility, especially when dealing with cancer. Last but not least, there are fabric dyes—most of which contain toxins—with which all cloth is made. Dark blue, brown, and black synthetic clothing may be more problematic insofar as laundering does not reverse a seemingly greater risk for contact dermatitis associated with that type of clothing.

Synthetic fabrics often are made with or from petro-chemicals. Natural fabrics, e.g., cotton, flax (linen), wool, and silk, are almost unheard today. However, even when you find them, they, too, are impregnated with finishing chemicals. With close to 8,000 chemicals used in clothing manufacture, what is a person to do? Here's what I do, have done for umpteen years, and encourage everyone—especially cancer patients—to do:

> Purchase clothing that can be laundered before wearing. Use only *natural plant-based* laundry detergents and never use dryer sheets that add chemicals into clothing while drying. Ever smell them, especially sheets and pillowcases one sleeps on for 6 to 8 hours a night? Whew!
>
> Into the washer rinse cycle add ¼ cup white distilled vinegar and *no* fabric softener.
>
> Dry either on a clothesline or preferably in a clothes dryer set on the highest heat setting the fabric can take,

which will 'bake or cook' out chemical residues, and *without* a dryer sheet.

For clothing that cannot be laundered, e.g., a new coat, I don't recommend dry cleaning as that only puts more petrochemicals into clothing. My suggestion is to place the garment into your clothes dryer at the highest heat setting for the longest time possible along with a wet washcloth that has been wrung out very well, not dripping wet. Moisture coming off the washcloth will act to push chemical fumes out the dryer exhaust. You may have to do that procedure for three or four cycles before new clothing chemicals are 'cooked' out of a garment that cannot be laundered. All natural and synthetic fabric garments can be 'cooked' in a dryer to release and vent toxic chemicals to the outdoors.

So what's a person to do about clothing choices? I suggest choosing natural fabrics and clothing made from:

- Cotton, preferably organically grown
- Linen, made from the flax plant
- Silk: Be aware it can be loaded with synthetic dyes
- Wool, preferably organically grown
- Other natural fibers: alpaca, angora, cashmere, mohair, and ramie—one of the oldest vegetable fibers from the nettle family of plants and thought to have been used by the ancient Egyptians.

Shoes, especially those made from rubber and plastic, can gas out terrible toxins into your living space. Be forewarned.

In the book, *Killer Clothes*, authors Anna Marie Clement and Brian R Clement talk about limiting bra wearing by females. Furthermore, there's the contention that restrictive bras suppress the lymphatic system's ability to flush toxins from breast tissue. You may recall in Chapter 23 I discussed the lymphatic system and suggested a certain type of brushing technique and massage to enhance lymphatic drainage of the breasts. Check out this web site for more information on bras and breast cancer <007b.com/bras_breast_cancer.php>.

Nightclothes, bedclothes, pajamas, nightgowns, etc. all should be loose fitting and 100 percent cotton so that your skin can 'breathe'. Never sleep wearing a bra. And last but not least, avoid under wire bras, as they can interfere with circulation and impact electromagnetic impulses coming out of the spinal column into the torso and chest. See Chapter 40, *Chiropractic & Cancer Management* for more information about that.

So, please keep this in mind, "Don't dress to kill."

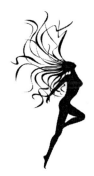

Chapter Thirty-One
Coffee and Cancer: What's the Connection?

Chocolate, men, coffee—some things are better rich.

… Anonymous

*J*ust about everyone appreciates a *cuppa Joe*. How do you like yours? Cream and sugar, black, black with sugar, milk and sugar, *Cappuccino, Espresso,* or *Latté?* How about an enema? Yes, an enema!

By the way, before we go any further on the coffee enema, and you think I've lost my marbles, I'd like to assure you that coffee enemas had been promoted in the **Merck Manual**, that prestigious repository of medical information, from the latter part of the nineteenth century (around 1890) in editions up until 1977. Do you believe that? I think a reason for deleting it may have been that they needed more space for modern scientific information. So why, then, does allopathy condemn coffee enemas as quackery when the *'mother'* of all medical information promoted coffee enemas for over three-quarters of a century?

Coffee may do more for your body as an enema than as a quick-picker-upper that gets you going in the morning. What coffee enemas do is to induce purging of the liver to release toxins that have been stored there from a lifetime of chemical exposure, and more recently from chemotherapy cancer treatments that, if not excreted from the body, probably will take their toll.

Perhaps by now you are thinking that I've lost it totally and there's nothing but bunk in this chapter, if not the book. Well, if you are one who believes your eyes, then maybe you ought to reserve any opinions until you check out *mucoid plaque* (also known as biofilm) at the Arise and Shine website at <ariseand-shine.com/mucoidplaque.aspx>. Please read *Plaque Facts*, then study the very graphic photograph of mucoid plaque. But before you watch the video, please pan down the page to read *Plaque Facts* and then study graphic photographs of mucoid plaque. I think you will have a different opinion about the immune system, much of which resides in the intestinal tract.

Before we consider coffee enemas further, maybe we ought to talk briefly about the physiology of toxicity from *a body's perspective*. That toxicity may have been accumulating over the years from lifestyle exposures to chemical toxins, tobacco use, alcoholic beverages, and toxic chemicals in daily food, plus incidental prescription drugs and vaccinations we may have taken.

Everything humans are exposed to has an impact upon the ecology of the body—the *"inner terrain"* as Beauchamp said—and must be eliminated and detoxified. Toxins can be found in air, water, food, cosmetics, the environment, work environments, medical procedures and medications, toxic amalgam and root canal dentistry—just to name a few. Even though we may not realize that toxic fumes and chemicals are taken into our bodies via breathing, eating, skin contact, and/or injection, they are. Our immune system and organs of detoxification—liver, kidneys, spleen to some extent, the skin via perspiration, and the colon—do Herculean jobs of removing many toxins from the body and we remain relatively healthy. However, when the body burden of toxins overloads, that's when diseases become apparent, and cancer in particular, since cancer is the manifestation of great toxic insult to the body. Coffee enemas, therefore, improve liver and gall bladder functions while removing toxic wastes from tumor breakdown, something allopathic cancer treatment really doesn't address and, unfortunately, leaves cancer patients toxic while continuing to add more chemotherapy.

So, for the sake of argument, let's agree that everyone has some toxic load within his or her body that's rattling around in there which triggers a cancer, breast cancer in particular. If a patient undergoes conventional allopathic treatments for breast cancer, there are all sorts of toxic chemicals called chemotherapy that are added to the body's already problematic toxic overload that led to the cancer in the first place. Depending upon what type of chemotherapy one takes—and none are exempt—the liver and kidneys are impacted big time. Please see Chapter 10, *Chemotherapy and Renal Failure.*

In addition to organ distress or failure, candida usually is ramping up big time in the body and overtaking the immune system. When candida gets into the bloodstream, that's not good. Medically it's called *Candida sepsis* and is extremely difficult to treat, often with fatal consequences. Patients don't want to get to that stage. Many cancer patients taking chemotherapy contract candida of the mouth or tongue—thrush, a very painful, toxic condition from chemotherapy.

Now let's get to the point of what coffee enemas have to do with all this. Many cancer patients who have had chemo and either have been told to go home and get their affairs in order, or have left the treatment regimen for whatever reason, wind up on the doorstep of holistic healthcare physicians. They need medical care and their oncologists have given up on them. They are so toxic that a most efficient way to start moving toxic chemicals and waste out of their body is to induce what is called a 'liver flush' utilizing the caffeine in coffee to encourage the liver to release toxins. And it works, but the regimen has to be monitored by a physician who understands that toxins cannot be moved out of the body too fast as the patient will feel very sick, and that can be scary. But those toxic poisons have to get out of the body, if one is to heal the cancer and the body.

In my opinion, that's where allopathic cancer treatment is lacking greatly. It has all these chemotherapy drugs that are designed to kill cancer cells but conventional oncology care and treatments do not give any thought to the huge amount of toxic waste matter that is accumulating within the patient's body and overloading the immune system. In essence, the average cancer patient taking chemotherapy is a toxic waste site, if you will pardon my saying that. Check out chemotherapy ingredient labels. Don't the treating technicians wear special protective clothing and gloves? How are the containers handled? As hazardous medical waste! If you don't believe that statement, I heartily recommend you check out the Wisconsin Department of Natural Resources Health Care Initiative Fact Sheet (PUB WA-1258 2008), "Managing Chemotherapy Waste."

The Fact Sheet lists the nine "Hazardous Waste Chemotherapy Drugs." Wow! And that stuff is pumped into your body! See if I'm exaggerating. Read it for yourself at <dnr.wi.gov/files/PDF/pubs/wa/wa1258.pdf>. Oh by the way, don't forget to check out the flow chart on that website.

Coffee enemas must be made with organically grown coffee and brewed with pure, non-fluoridated water. There is a special regimen to follow that a holistic physician provides and which I will not go into here. That's not my intent. My encouragement is that you seek out proper instructions, guidance, and monitoring while taking a course of coffee enema treatments, if that's your desire. Please do NOT do it on your own without proper guidance, especially if you have had chemotherapy.

Before you think coffee is the only enema ingredient, the herb chamomile made into a tea also can be used as a bowel cleanse. Chamomile also can be used as a body soak, which can help induce relaxation before bedtime.

As with any natural, chemical, pharmaceutical, or vaccine ingredient(s), be on the lookout for allergic reactions, especially when ingested or injected.

Again, my most sincere advice is to seek the counsel and guidance of a qualified holistic medical doctor who can guide you.

It's tea for two, but a coffee enema for one.

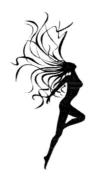

Chapter Thirty-Two
Sleep: What Does It Have to Do With Breast Cancer?

This is the great error of our day in the treatment of the human body, that physicians separate the soul from the body.

... Hippocrates (c.460BCE—370BCE)
The Father of Modern Medicine

*M*any scientists—metaphysically oriented ones in particular—feel that during sleep our consciousness 'travels' to other dimensions where we get re-energized. Numerous cultures have believed in dreams—the Assyrians, Babylonians, Egyptians, Greeks, and Romans—which, apparently back then and now, are considered an integral component of sleep. There's even a discipline of sorts known as dream interpretation. Does that make sense? Only in retrospect do dreamers sometimes relate to what a dream may have been foretelling.

In the Old Testament of the Bible we hear stories of famous dreamers and their dreams, e.g.,

- Jacob's beautiful dream at Bethel of a ladder of angels ascending into heaven;
- Joseph, the youngest of twelve brothers and his beautiful multi-color coat, who could interpret dreams and told of famine years to come;
- Daniel who could interpret dreams like no one before or since;
- King Solomon, considered the wisest person to have lived;
- Job talks about how dreams teach and instruct during sleep.

And in the New Testament,

- Joseph, the husband of Mary the mother of Jesus, was told in a dream to take the Baby and His mother into Egypt until called back by instructions through another dream.

Admittedly, there are those who regard dreams as 'evil divinations' that scare dreamers or those folks who don't know about or how to interact with a part of one's psyche that deals with the unknown, often referred to as metaphysics or spirituality—not religion. We have a certain energy within us that can only be proven by what is termed death. One minute a human body is functional or near functional and the next, the body is here but it cannot do a thing. The life breath is gone; *chi* has departed. That is the aspect of spirituality that I'm talking about; some call it the soul; others, spirit; and a few, nothing.

So really, what do sleep and dreams have to do with breast cancer, you ask? First, we have to grasp that our bodies and biological functions operate on a *circadian rhythm,* which basically means according to a set or specific time of day. Oriental medicine considers that aspect of human biochemistry in much more detail.

The pineal gland in the brain secretes melatonin, known as the "hormone of darkness." Melatonin also can be produced in bone marrow cells, lymphocytes, and epithelial cells. Why such a strange nickname? Because it 'regulates' the sleep process during the *dark hours* of the day when humans normally are expected *by Nature to sleep* and recharge adrenal glands and the body in general.

When people are deprived of quality sleep *at night*—or even sleep with a light on—the body reacts by producing low levels of melatonin. Strangely, the reduced levels of melatonin have been considered as contributing to higher rates of cancer in night shift workers.

Furthermore, melatonin is being investigated as a radio-protective agent from free radical damage caused by ionizing radiation. Cancer radiation therapy emits ionizing radiation. (Read Chapter 9, *Radiation: What Is It?)* So how does melatonin impact breast cancer?

According to published research by Gonzalez A, et al. "Melatonin promotes differentiation of 3T3-L1 fibroblasts" in the *Journal of Pineal Research*, May 26, 2011,

> *Melatonin inhibits the genesis and growth of breast cancer by interfering at different levels in the estrogen-signaling pathways. Melatonin inhibits aromatase activity and*

expression in human breast cancer cells, thus behaving as a selective estrogen enzyme modulator. ... These findings suggest that, in human breast tumors, melatonin could stimulate the differentiation of fibroblasts and reduce the aromatase activity and expression in both fibroblasts and adipocytes, thereby reducing the number of estrogen-producing cells proximal to malignant cells. [114]

In another published study by Lee SL, et al. "MicroRNA and gene expression analysis of melatonin-exposed human breast cancer cell lines indicating involvement of the anticancer effect" in the *Journal of Pineal Research*, April 21, 2011,

Furthermore, melatonin is reported to have an anticancer function including suppression of the metabolism of tumor cells and induction of tumor suppressor genes in cancer cells, including breast cancer cells. ... Our findings suggested that melatonin may modulate miRNA and gene expression as an anticancer mechanism in human breast cancer cells. [115]

Blask DE, et al. in their published study "Circadian regulation of molecular, dietary, and metabolic signaling mechanisms of human breast cancer growth by the nocturnal melatonin signal and the consequences of its disruption by light at night" published April 2, 2011 in the *Journal of Pineal Research*, state,

This review article discusses recent work on the melatonin-mediated circadian regulation and integration of

molecular, dietary, and metabolic signaling mechanisms involved in human breast cancer growth and the consequences of circadian disruption by exposure to light at night (LAN). Experimental evidence in rats and humans indicating that LAN-induced circadian disruption of the nocturnal melatonin signal activates human breast cancer growth, metabolism, and signaling provides the strongest mechanistic support, thus far, for population and ecological studies demonstrating elevated breast cancer risk in night shift workers and other individuals increasingly exposed to LAN. [116]

And, a study published in May 2011 indicates that higher risks of breast and endometrial cancers have been associated with female night shift workers. So *sleeping at night* is very important to human physiology, it seems. That being said, research also indicates that melatonin inhibits aromatase, an enzyme that makes estradiol and other estrogens in women—and men too. When estradiol is inhibited there seems to be an impact on breast cancer via anti-estrogenic activity.

What recent research seems to be indicating is that a lack of melatonin is correlated with an increase in breast cancer risks. But men also should take note since Japanese research indicates that melatonin can suppress prostate cancer.

Taking supplements can increase melatonin. I heartily recommend a good night's sleep for various reasons. I suggest your discussing melatonin supplementation with your physician before embarking on a self-help protocol. Studies have indicated it's safe. Many people take melatonin about thirty minutes before bedtime to get a good night's sleep instead of taking a sleeping pill. One indicator of a good night's sleep is called REM sleep. That's often when we find ourselves in dreamland. Rapid Eye Movement sleep occurs several times during a night's sleeping pattern. Our most vivid dreams usually occur then.

Keeping our body's natural circadian rhythms according to Mother Nature's clock may be an unknown in dealing with and curing breast cancer.

Oh to sleep, perchance to dream—forget the nightmares.

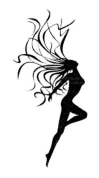

Chapter Thirty-Three
Off-the-Wall Stuff

*The only way to keep your health is to eat what you don't want,
drink what you don't like, and do what you'd rather not.*

...Samuel L Clemens aka Mark Twain (1835—1910)
American author & humorist

Mr Clemens, your humor was 'dry' at times, like this.

As the title of this chapter suggests, you will read about suggestions that may not make sense to you for whatever reason, but I propose that you seriously consider the information, as it may—and can—affect your overall well being and ability to get well.

Please keep in mind that some of the *wisdom* being imparted just may take a while to sink in and be 'digested' before you can appreciate its value.

- Chew or masticate each mouthful of food a minimum of twenty (20) times before swallowing. Food needs to be ensalivated with enzymes in saliva to start the digestive process that winds its way through the 'labyrinth' it must take to ensure your body's cells get vital nutrients. To see all that's involved, I suggest visiting <innerbody.com/image/digeov.html>.

- Discontinue wearing battery-operated wristwatches or carrying or wearing any battery-operated device on your body. There's a theory that batteries interfere with meridians and *chi* flowing in the body—for what it's worth.

- Definitely discontinue wearing a 'live-active' cell phone on your body because of electromagnetic radiation. See this website for the reasons <emf-health.com/articles-10tips.htm>.

- Limit your time before a computer terminal at least until you stabilize. I turn off the printer when working at the computer and turn on the printer only when I need to print something.

- Stay a least 8-10 feet away from an operating TV set.

- Keep a clock radio alarm clock at least 3 feet away from your head in bed.

- Stay out of a microwave oven's wavelength when the door is opened after it's been operating. Radiation wavelengths escape.

- **No microwave cooked food for cancer patients.** *Micro waved food may contain both molecules and energies not present in food cooked in the way humans have*

been cooking food since they discovered how to cook food.
Visit online <herbalhealer.com/microwave.html>.

- Microwave heated water apparently causes problems for plants watered with it. Check out <rawhealthyyou. com/2011/02/02/microwaved-water-that-kills-plants-what-does-it-do-to-humans/>.

- Eliminate as much exposure to electronic radiation as possible, such as cordless phones, computer games, tanning beds, cell phones, etc.

- Airplane travel for frequent flyers: Something to consider—geomagnetic energy and radiation, in addition to ionizing radiation from the TSA scanners at check in. Check out this website <forbiddenknowledgetv.com/ videos/earth-sciences/geomagnetic-conspiracy— part-2.html>.

Society has been acculturated through advertising, television, books, magazines, media spin, and family physicians to revere everything medical as if it truly were a 'gift from the gods'. However and sad to say, those medical 'gifts' often turn into something more than double edged swords. Both medical and media literature chronicle drug recalls and class action suits for medical paraphernalia and prescription drugs that have damaged humans. Vaccines are exempt; Big Pharma is going wild creating many more so that there will be no financial or product liability from prescription drugs gone awry in the future when vaccines replace Rxs, I think. In my opinion, Big Pharma is gearing up to produce a vaccine to 'prevent' even hangnails, that's how prolific vaccinology will become down the road within the next ten years, maybe sooner. Can't blame them, I guess, since Congress gave them *carte blanche*.

However, Big Pharma had to pay the piper plenty because menopausal drugs have caused breast cancer in three Pennsylvania women. Pfizer Inc. must pay $72.6 million to three women who took such drugs as *Premarin*®, *Provera*®, and *Prempro*®, all manufactured by subsidiaries of Pfizer, one of—if not—the largest research and pharmaceutical manufacturers in the world.

The moral of that legal outcome, I think, is women should learn how to take care of their bodies throughout their reproductive years so that menopause can be 'a breeze'. I know; I went through it without a hot flash and didn't even know it. Taking synthetic hormones is like playing Russian roulette, I think. But then, as I said, women—like everyone else—are acculturated to believe there is magic in those artificial hormones. The 'magic' is that years later, something else you don't want, usually pops up like a rabbit out of a magician's hat, as the three Pennsylvania ladies found out, and it was breast cancer.

Truth sometimes really can be funnier than fiction.

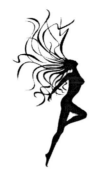

Chapter Thirty-Four
Holistic PREVENTIVE Measures To Avoid Breast Cancer

The man [or woman] who never alters his [or her] opinion is like standing water, and breeds reptiles of the mind.

… William Blake (1757—1827)
English poet

Everything you've read so far, hopefully, makes sense to your deep feelings and growing awareness. Much of the information probably has been innovative but documented, and I hope exciting to learn.

I can remember telling folks all my life who questioned how I know what I know, that I didn't come out of my mother's womb knowing what I know now. I had to seek the information, which eventually led to a storehouse of holistic health knowledge. That zeal and subsequent quest came from almost being killed by the medical profession while a young woman. The only way I can describe it is you just know what's right for you and what's not; then you seek to become educated where your heart and conscience take you.

I've learned that others may be able to fool me, but they can't fool my body; it knows when it can't handle chemicals and toxins wherever they may appear in today's modern lifestyle. I don't think I'm unique. What I do think is unique about me is that I have connected dots from studies and research, etc. to the place where I understand that man-made chemicals really are not the 'saving grace' of modern life. They are contributing to our health's downfall, I believe.

So, how does one really go about avoiding breast cancer, or any form of cancer? Where shall we start?

For parents who are concerned about their children

I suggest learning about the neurotoxins and other poisons in vaccines that are touted as safe. Nothing can be further from scientific fact since formaldehyde, Formalin, mercury, aluminum, foreign DNA, aborted human fetus cells (diploid cells), viruses, and an entire roster of chemicals with industrial uses are used in the manufacture of vaccines. Don't want to believe that? How about checking out the CDC's official site for ***Vaccine Excipient & Media Summary*** at <cdc.gov/vaccines/pubs/pinkbook/downloads/appendices/b/excipient-table-1.pdf>.

Carefully study the list and then do some research online about the chemicals you find in the CDC's listing. Also, you may want to read some of my articles published at <vactruth.com>.

As you read in Chapter 7, *Whom or What Can We Trust*, there was SV40 and cancer in the polio vaccine that was injected into millions of people that Congress admits no one knows how many contracted cancer from that fiasco. *Long-range health effects from vaccines literally are unknown territory* even though we know some of the immediate and short range devastating health problems for children.

Allergy 'Hallmarks' To Recognize

From what I know of body chemistry, there are some sign-posts along the way that can clue you as to how your body is faring and what to do to prevent health problems.

- *Do you have allergies?* If yes, that's indication that your immune system is stressed, not working efficiently, and probably being triggered when it should not. Allergies, in my opinion, need to be tended to, and that usually means removing toxins (detox programs) from the body and strengthening the immune system with nutrient rich, organically grown—*no GMO foods*—and a change of lifestyle from one that's embedded in chemicals, e.g., bug sprays, pet flea dips, chemical lawn care, scented products, fluoridated water, tobacco products, etc. I suggest your reading my 2009 book *Our Chemical Lives And The Hijacking Of Our DNA, A Probe Into What's Probably Making Us Sick.*
- *Do you experience dark circles either around or beneath your eyes?* In holistic health parlance, these euphemistically are referred to as 'allergy shiners' and show up after eating an allergen. However, many folks

unknowingly eat offending foods daily and, consequently, have permanent 'black eyes' that they think
may be normal for them. Dark circles around the eyes
also can indicate low thyroid function.

Body Ecology Issues

- *Do you have fungus in or on your body?* Do you have
  ringworm? Are your toenails or fingernails thick, yellow,
  and crusty with fungus growth? Such growth also could be
  ringworm of the nail, dermatophytes, molds, candida, or
  even a nail bed tumor. With toenails or fingernails sport-
  ing such 'crustiness' your body probably is a host to some
  sort of parasite that not only is living off of you, but also is
  depositing its metabolic wastes into your bloodstream and
  that isn't good. One could say that your body is a waste disposal or septic system for whatever is living off your body.
- *Do you have intestinal parasites?* Most folks do and
  don't know it, especially if you eat rare-cooked meats or
  raw fish or seafood. Children often get small pinworms
  from pets. There's the theory that once infested, you
  really can't get rid of them. I don't think that's factual,
  but if one has had intestinal parasites, one always should
  be vigilant to make certain the critters have not grown
  into a community again in your intestinal tract where
  they can form boluses and cause impactions. I've heard
  of worms in other organs of the body too. Parasites
  of any type live off your body and deposit their waste
  into your bloodstream. They go potty in you! Intestinal

parasites have cyclical patterns for reproduction that are important to know in order to deal with getting rid of them. There are many holistic approaches that are not based in toxic chemicals that will eliminate them. Seeing a holistic physician is the best way to deal with them. Your health will improve dramatically.

- *Have you taken antibiotics often or regularly?* Antibiotics ruin the ecological balance in the gut and intestinal tract. Even when antibiotics are absolutely necessary, probiotics should be taken with any course of antibiotics to preserve the integrity of intestinal flora.
- *Have you taken birth control pills?* They are one of the factors that I personally believe have had an impact upon breast cancer rates spiraling over the years, especially for young women, because of women using them without realizing how they impact female hormones and the 'games they play in female bodies'.
- *Do you have a vaginal discharge?* If so, that probably indicates a yeast (*Candida Albicans*) infection, which suppresses the immune system.
- *Do you wear panty liners because your vagina 'sweats'?*
- *In males, a comparable is jock itch.*

Food Issues and/or Concerns to Consider
- *Do you drink soda daily?* If so, you are feeding an entire population of microorganisms that live in acidic conditions, 'fertilized' by sugar, especially cancer cells.

- ***What's your daily sugar intake from all food?*** If you are eating pastries, candies, and other sugary foods, you are jeopardizing your body's pH balance that could lead to cancer cells forming. Sugar is *the* food of cancer cells, and anything that converts into sugar during digestion, e.g., high glycemic foods like bread, pizza, chips, pretzels, beer, alcohol, etc.

- ***Does your diet consist mainly of processed foods?*** They provide very little nutrients—and no enzymes—for the mitochondria in each of the 100 trillion cells in your body. What about your body's ability to healthfully maintaining 206 bones, 600 muscles, and 22 internal organs? What about GMO foods that contain 'unknowns'? What about all the free radicals that form during the digestive process from eating all the food preservatives, colors, and other food processing chemicals? How about free radicals from deep-fried and charbroiled foods?

- ***Do you drink rbST/rGBH hormone laced cows' milk?*** If you drink *non*-organically-produced milk and eat cheese, yogurt, ice cream and other dairy products made from it, you probably are ingesting recombinant DNA hormone-produced milk, which just may increase your chances or risks for breast cancer. Milk-producing hormones, some of which are injected daily into cows at the base of their tails to produce more milk, have been found to be residual in milk together with pus and antibiotics, which just may increase your chances and risks for breast cancer by promoting conversion of normal breast tissue into cancer cells. Those milk-producing hormones are banned in all European Union countries, Australia, Canada, and Japan. USA dairy products aren't imported in those countries because of rGBH. To understand more about that, please visit online <youtube .com/watch?v=3SXVpvgXo9Q>.

According to the warning label for
Monsanto's Posilac drug (their brand name for rBGH) explicitly states: "Cows injected with POSILAC are at an increased risk for clinical mastitis (visibly abnormal milk). The number of cows affected with clinical mastitis and the number of cases per cow may increase.... In some herds, use of POSILAC has been associated with increases in somatic cell counts [pus & bacteria]." The warning label goes on to say "use of POSILAC may result in an increase in digestive disorders such as indigestion, bloat, and diarrhea.... Studies indicated that cows injected with POSILAC had increased numbers of enlarged hocks and lesions (e.g., lacerations, enlargements, calluses) of the knee...and...of the foot region." [117]
Note: Pharmaceutical giant Eli Lilly acquired Monsanto's Posilac® [genetically engineered cow hormone] in 2008.

John Robbins, author of *The New Good Life: Living Better Than Ever in an Age of Less,* wrote this article August 10, 2010 for *HuffingtonPost*, "Female Infants Growing Breasts: Another Disaster From Hormones in Milk Production."

———

Instead of boring you with my words, please check it out for yourself online at <huffingtonpost.com/john-robbins/female-infants-growing-br_b_676402.html>

China and the USA both use bovine growth hormones.

- ***Do you smoke or chew tobacco?*** If so, you definitely may be inviting not only some form of cancer but also numerous other diseases to form in your body.

Lifestyle Issues

- ***Do you live in a 'healthy' house?*** Are your laundry detergents and household cleaning agents ecologically friendly and 'green'? Are you 'hooked' on ambient odors from scented products like candles and electrical outlet devices, which out gas potentially cancer causing chemical fumes that you constantly breathe? If you want to understand indoor air pollution, I suggest reading Chapter 18 *Indoor Pollution: More Serious Than You May Think* in my last book, *Our Chemical Lives And The Hijacking Of Our DNA, A Probe Into What's Probably Making Us Sick,* available on Amazon.com.

- ***Are you exposed to chemicals every night because you sleep on a mattress that's impregnated with fire retardant chemicals?*** Infants, children, and adults are exposed to and breathe those awful chemicals. There are organic and naturally safer bedroom, bath, lifestyle, and pet products available. Seven years ago I purchased my organic mattress and box spring from *Lifekind*

(<lifekind.com>) and could not be happier with both their product(s) and customer service.

- ***If you wear rubber or plastic sole shoes, maybe you ought to become familiar*** with the work of James Oschman, PhD, and his two books, *Energy Medicine: The Scientific Basis* and *Energy Medicine in Therapeutics and Human Performance.* Dr Oschman investigated grounding and how human connection to the earth can improve the quality of life such as reducing inflammation in the body, a cause of chronic disease including cancer. Oschman claims when one is grounded free electrons from earth transfer into the human body. Furthermore, he says that free electrons probably are the most potent antioxidants. One thing I'd like to caution about is coming in contact with pesticides sprayed on lawns or walkways when walking barefoot.

What To Do As Preventative Measures

- ***If you haven't seen a physician in a while, please get a physical and a comprehensive blood panel done NOW.*** That is the first line of defense, especially if you are looking to avoid cancer.
- ***If you are a female who has a family history of breast cancer, or any cancer,*** you will want to be especially vigilant with self-breast examinations and periodic checkups via *certain blood tests* that are *more accurate* than mammograms and don't give you ionizing radiation, and can detect cancer cells in the body.

Those blood tests are Tumor Markers:
  Cancer Antigen 15-3 (CA 15-3)
  Cancer Antigen 27-29 (CA 27-29).

Dr Lynn Morales recommends taking a CA 15-3 blood test every three to four months for those who are concerned, are borderline, or have family history of cancer. Those blood tests don't put ionizing radiation into your body like mammograms do.

There's another blood test that diagnoses specific cancers in the body, it's CA-125 (cancer or carbohydrate antigen).

Although this blood test is the one most often used as an ovarian cancer marker, it also is used to diagnose and track breast, endometrium, fallopian tube, gastrointestinal tract, and lung cancers.

- **Consider getting a Thermogram of both breasts as soon as possible to have a baseline reading.** It is FDA-approved with no ionizing radiation. Thermography photographs the heat coming off your body. Cancer cells produce heat, which specialized cameras can photograph. See Chapter 45, *Thermography.*
- *If you are taking birth control pills, maybe you ought to consider some other form of birth control that does not include synthetic pharmaceutical chemicals impacting hormones.* Some birth control pills combine synthetic hormones [ethinyl estradiol and norethindrone]. For more information about birth control

pills and a breast cancer connection, please visit this web site <ditchthepill.org/breastcancer.htm>.

In October 2006 the Mayo Clinic had this to say:

"Use of oral contraceptives is associated with an increased risk of pre-menopausal breast cancer, especially with use before FTTP (first full term pregnancy) in parous women (women who have given birth)."

- ***Introduce antioxidants into your diet via food, tea, and supplements.*** I think drinking a detoxifying herbal tea daily is helpful, especially one that promotes healthy liver function like *Traditional Medicinals Lemon EveryDay Detox,* which contains organically grown burdock root, stinging nettle leaf, cleavers herb, dandelion root, and lemon myrtle leaf.

- ***Stop alcohol consumption.*** Research studies indicate that drinking three to six alcoholic beverages a week can increase a female's chances for contracting breast cancer. Several studies results confirming that connection are published in *JAMA,* the *Journal of the American Medical Association.* Again, I point you to an online website so that you can get a better understanding of the issue. Please see <jama.ama-assn.org/search?fulltext=alcohol+ and+breast+cancer&submit=yes&x=13&y=8>.

- ***Reduce red meat consumption from daily to twice a week and to organically grown meats from cattle not raised on synthetic hormones to fatten them.*** Here's a website that lists supermarkets selling grass-fed, pasture raised animal meat brands. <humaneitarian.org/

where-do-i-buy-humanelyraised-meat/grocery-stores/
your-supermarket/>.

- *Change your diet immediately to one that imitates the diet suggested in this book. Eat plenty green vegetables daily, especially those from the cabbage or cole family. Introduce fresh garlic into your cooking. It's a natural fungicide found in food.*
- *The quickest, easiest, and most non-toxic ways to adjust body chemistry are to change to organically grown food, a diet free of sugar, and non-fluoridated water.*
- *Eliminate stress from your life. Learn to say "NO" especially to those who take you for granted, which often happens in relationships and life.*
- *Give yourself some TLC every day no matter how busy you are. Take time to go within and find your inner gyroscope that is waiting there to be rediscovered and worked with.*

Alternative or Holistic Health Modalities You May Want To Consider

After all you have read in this book, and this chapter in particular, you probably are thinking what does conventional medicine think about holistic health treatments. Well, are you ready for this? None other than the prestigious Mayo Clinic has this to say about alternative cancer treatments:

Alternative cancer treatments won't play any role in curing your cancer, but they may help you cope with signs and symptoms caused by cancer and cancer treatments.

Common signs and symptoms such as anxiety, fatigue, nausea and vomiting, pain, difficulty sleeping, and stress may be lessened by alternative treatments. [118]

Even though Mayo Clinic may not think nor agree that alternative cancer treatments can cure cancer—which, of course, they do, and happens all the time, just do your research—Mayo does say alternative treatments may help cancer patients cope with what are recognized as problems that may be originating from conventional cancer treatments.

However, I specifically omitted "*may help you cope with signs and symptoms caused by cancer.*" Did you catch that? Isn't that tacit admission or a back door endorsement that alternative or holistic health modalities work, i.e., help a cancer patient to cope? Where are the coping modalities within conventional oncology? Even biofeedback, which some utilize, came out of complementary and alternative medicine (CAM).

Too many patients have gone the conventional cancer treatment route only to receive a "can't do any more for you" let down and then do find help—and even cures—in holistic cancer management.

The Mayo Clinic web site shows a chart listing symptoms for which a cancer patient can use alternative treatments, which includes acupuncture, aromatherapy, biofeedback, exercise, hypnosis, massage, meditation, music therapy, relaxation techniques, tai chi, and yoga to help in finding relief or how to cope. Personally, I want to thank Mayo for their willingness to place that important information on their web site. I truly believe the Mayo Clinic truly is providing a great service to cancer patients by doing that. Again, I congratulate them for their willingness to extend a hand of friendship toward alternative/holistic medicine and a recognition that it does work. I wish others were as progressive and 'ecumenical' as Mayo Clinic is in its thinking about CAM.

However, missing from Mayo's recommendations is the key to battling cancer, in my opinion, and that is changing body chemistry via a totally natural and organic diet— something that may be anathema to conventional medicine since it is steeped in hospital-type food service and chemicals, i.e., chemotherapy and prescription drugs, plus all foods are chemicalized either in the fields—including GMOs, or during processing, with the exception of organics that food processors now want to contaminate with exceptions to organic labeling rules.

I sincerely believe the best and most effective route for dealing with any cancer, and breast cancer in particular, is to change body chemistry as quickly and as efficiently as possible to stop cancer cells from metastasizing and to promote apoptosis—cancer cell suicide.

When body pH maintains 7.4 cancer cells are 'dormant'; when body pH reaches 8.4, cancer cells die off (apoptosis). A diet high in pH value, as discussed in this book, will achieve that more quickly than you realize, especially when raw green juices are used. That is key in winning the war on cancer, I truly believe, as additional chemicals in the body only cause more problems for the breast cancer patient to deal with, and as the Mayo Clinic's web site accurately states, *"signs and symptoms caused by cancer and cancer treatments."*

There definitely is more than one way to do anything and/or achieve results. Why allopathic medicine contends holistic cancer treatments don't work is just plain bunk, and part of its public relations spin control campaign, I think. Remember what Special Counsel Fitzgerald found out in 1953 regarding cancer treatments? I think that has to stop and both camps in healthcare need to work together without allopathy maintaining its 'top dog' and predatory status. That's when women *will win* the war on *breast* cancer.

Don't worry! Enjoy life and be grateful for what you have, including those things that annoy you. They are there to teach lessons.

Believe in the miracles of life and living; they truly are wonderful and empowering.

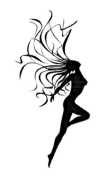

Chapter Thirty-Five
Information Resources

Knowledge is power.

… **Sir Francis Bacon (1561—1626)**
English author & philosopher

Reports

Breast Cancer Cover-up ISBN 978-1-4507-6201-4

Buried Treatments that are Wiping Out Tumors When Nothing Else Will

Authors: Lee Euler with Susan Clark

Publisher: Online Publishing & Marketing, LLC, PO Box 1076, Lexington, VA 24450

Bonus Report: **Your Breast Cancer Action Plan**

What to Do if You Get Breast Cancer (2011)
Same authors and publisher as above.

Cancer Breakthrough USA! ISBN 978-1-4243-4496-3

Authors: Frank Cousineau with Andrew Scholberg

345

Publisher: Online Publishing & Marketing, LLC, PO Box 1076, Lexington, VA 24450

Fight Cancer and Win! (a free e-book offered by Michael Cutler, MD)

Author: Michael Cutler, MD, Editor

Publisher: Easy Health Options, LLC, PO Box 3703, Hueytown, AL 35023

<easyhealthoptions.com>Phone: 1-800-523-5593

How to Cure Almost Any Cancer at Home for $5.15 a Day ISBN 978-1-61539-952-9

Authors: Bill Henderson with Andrew Scholberg

Publisher: Online Publishing & Marketing, LLC, PO Box 1076, Lexington, VA 24450

How to Cure Almost Any Cancer at Home online link

<haturalcancerremedies.com/515/09120PM.html>

<naturalcancerremedies.com/31D/1205EHO2.html>

Natural Strategies for Cancer Patients

Author: Russell Blaylock, MD

Publisher: <blaylockwellnesscenter.com>

Today's Greatest Alternative Medicines

Authors: The Research Staff at Health Sciences Institute

Publisher: Institute of Health Sciences, LLC, 819 N. Charles St., Baltimore, MD 21201 (Phone: 630-236-4653)

Books

Cancer – Step Outside The Box 5th Edition ISBN 0-9788065-0-6

Author: Ty M Bolinger

Publisher: Infinity 510 Squared Partners

Healing Outside the Margins ISBN 0-89526-193-6

The Survivor's Guide to Integrative Cancer Care

Authors: Carole O'Toole with Carolyn B. Hendricks, MD, Medical Advisor

Publisher: LifeLine Press, Washington, DC

Heal Yourself ISBN 13:978-1-934716-23-6

Author: Dr Lynne Zimmerman

Publisher: Sunrise River Press

Knockout ISBN 978-0-307-58746-6

Interviews with Doctors Who Are Curing Cancer and How to Prevent Getting It In the First Place

Author: Suzanne Somers

Publisher: Crown Publishers, division of Random House, New York City

Outsmart Your Cancer 2nd Edition ISBN 978-0-9728867-8-9

Alternative Non-Toxic Treatments That Work

Author: Tanya Harter Pierce

Publisher: Thought Works Publishing, Stateline, Nevada

Pocket Guide To MACROBIOTICS ISBN 978-0-89594-848-9
Author: Carl Ferré In cooperation with the George Ohsawa Macrobiotic Foundation
Publisher: Crossing Press, Berkeley / Toronto

Recaging The Beast ISBN 978-0-9830311-0-9
The Disease Behind Disease: The Yeast-Fungal Connection
Author: Jane Remington
Publisher: Obsidian Press

The Cancer Prevention Diet ISBN 978-0-312-56106-2
The Macrobiotic Approach to Preventing and Relieving Cancer
Authors: Michio Kushi and Alex Jack
Publisher: St Martin's Griffin, New York

The Encyclopedia of Medical Breakthroughs & Forbidden Treatments ISBN 978-0-9749859-3-0
Health Secrets and Little-Known Therapies For Specific Health Conditions From A-to-Z
Author: Medical Research Associates, LLC
Publisher: Medical Research Associates, LLC, PO Box 55725, Seattle, WA 98155

The Healing Consciousness ISBN 0-9766678-4-3
A Doctor's Journey to Healing
Author: Beth Baughman DuPree, MD
Publisher: WovenWord Press, 811 Mapleton Ave., Boulder, CO 80304

The Secret History of the WAR on CANCER ISBN 978-0-465-01566-5

Author: Devra Davis, PhD, MPH
Publisher: Basic Books, A Member of the Perseus Books Group, New York

The Yeast-Free Kitchen ISBN 1-41200797-6
Recipes To Help You Achieve Victory Over The Yeast-Beast, Candida Albicans
Author: Jane Remington
Publisher: Trafford Publishing, Ste. 6E, 2333 Government St., Victoria, BC, V8T 4P4, Canada

Tomorrow's Cancer Cures Today ISBN 978-1-891434-41-9
25 Secret Therapies from around the world
Author: Allan Spreen, MD
Publisher: Health Sciences Institute, Baltimore, Maryland

DVDs / Videos / Movies

Burzynski The Movie - Cancer Is Serious Business [1 hr 45 minutes DVD]
Publisher: ME Rola
More Information: <burzynskimovie.com>

Cancer Is Curable NOW
<canceriscurablenow.tv/buy-now>

Holistic Health Institute: Greatest New Medicines of Our Time

<hsionlineorders.net/video/ACS_OLP/?pco=E6DDM
CCI&efo=HSIOP02&o=539243&s=543206&u=490
01557&l=342591&g=84&r=Milo>

Publisher: Holistic Health Institute

**How I Cured Myself Of Breast Cancer With No Drugs
And No Surgery**

Author: Susan Insole

Publisher: Holistic Voice <holisticvoice.org/BreastCancer
Cured.html>

**One Answer To Cancer They Don't Want You To Know
About...**

Author/Producer: Elaine Hollingsworth

Publisher: <OneAnswerToCancerMovie.com>

Why Food Matters

Author: Ana Sofia Joanes

Publisher: Fresh
<org2.democracyinaction.org/o/5958/p/d/freshthe-
movie/shop/itemDetail.sjs?store_item_KEY=1842>

Inspirational and Meditation Tapes

Angel Therapy Meditations [Compact Disc] ISBN
978-1-4019-1832-3

Author: Doreen Virtue, PhD

Publisher: HayHouse Body-Mind-Spirit

Positive Imagery For People With Cancer [cassette tape]

Side A: The Healing Image

Side B: Targeting Your Treatment
Author: Emmett E Miller, MD
Publisher: <drmiller.com>
The Patient Package [Compact Disc]
Includes: 2 Books: *Getting Well Again & The Healing Journey*
2 CDs: *Getting Well*
Author: Emmett E Miller, MD
Publisher:
Relaxation & Mental Imagery as Applies to Cancer Therapy
Available: <simontoncenter.com/proddetail.asp?prod=120>
Phone: 800-338-2360

Holistic Health Newsletters
Cancer Defeated [Archived issues on file]
<cancerdefeatedpublications.com/main_folder/newsletters/>
To Subscribe
<cancerdefeatedpublications.com/newsletters/signup.html>

Easy Health Options ™
To Subscribe
<subscriptions@easyhealthoptions.com>
Mercola.com Newsletter / Joseph Mercola, DO
To Subscribe

<articles.mercola/subscribe.aspx>
The Blaylock Wellness Report **Living A Long Healthy Life / Russell L Blaylock, MD**
To Subscribe
<blaylockreport.com>
Townsend Letter **The Examiner of Alternative Medicine / Jonathan V Wright, MD**
To Subscribe
<townsendletter.com/subscriptions.htm>

Holistic Cruises at Sea
Annual Vegan Cruises with Christina Pirello of *PBS TV show "Christina Cooks"*
Details: <atasteofhealth.org>
Phone: 800-496-0989

Christina Pirello's Cooking Intensive on Macrobiotic Cruise 2
Video showing Christina's natural vegetarian cooking class at sea
<youtube.com/watch?v=3BGZM_XbTEc>
Christina on Breast Cancer
<youtube.com/watch?v=RngEvWn-rC4&feature=youtube_gdata_player>
Christina's Story: Cured of Leukemia at Age 26 using Macrobiotic diet
<christinacooks.com/my_story>

Holistic Holiday at Sea *offered by A Taste of Health, Coral Gables, Florida*

Phone: 828-749-9537

Website: <atasteofhealth.org>

Pampering Cruise, Healthy Natural Cuisine, Enlightening Seminars and Workshops

One never can know enough about some things.

Part III
Holistic Non-Toxic Healthcare Resources

"The doctor of the future will give no medicine, but will interest her or his patients in the care of the human frame, in a proper diet, and in the cause and prevention of disease."

Thomas A Edison
American Inventor 1847—1931

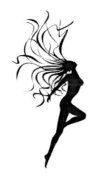

Chapter Thirty-Six
Integrative Cancer Care
Holistic-Conventional Treatment
Facilities for Cancer

Never, never, never give up.

… Sir Winston Churchill (1874—1965)
British statesman

For cancer patients who want a more holistic approach but one that encompasses conventional allopathic cancer treatments, e.g., surgery-radiation-chemotherapy, ***Cancer Treatment Centers of America*** (CTCA) just may be what you are looking for.

CTCA hospitals staffs include surgical oncologists, radiation oncologists, gastroenterologists, urologists, intake physicians, naturopathic physicians, mind-body therapists, nutritionists, chiropractors, acupuncturists, pastoral care staff, and oncology rehabilitation.

To investigate Cancer Treatment Options at CTCA, visit their website at <cancercenter.com/cancer-treatments.cfm>

Most health insurance plans pay for cancer treatment at CTCA. However, HMOs do not cover cancer treatment at CTCA. For individual coverage information, it would be wise—and I suggest—for you to talk with your healthcare insurance provider first or contact:

Cancer Treatment Centers of America
Phone: 800-615-3055 Online: <cancercenter.com>
To Discuss Treatment Options
800-931-9299

Eastern Regional Medical Center
Cancer Treatment & Wellness Center
1331 East Wyoming Avenue
Philadelphia, PA 19124
Online: <cancercenter.com/eastern-hospital.cfm>
Phone: 215-537-7400

Midwestern Regional Medical Center
Cancer Treatment & Wellness Center
2520 Elisha Avenue
Zion, IL 60099 (suburban Chicago)
Online: <cancercenter.com/midwestern-hospital.cfm>
Phone: 847-872-4561

Seattle Cancer Treatment & Wellness Center
Cancer Treatment & Wellness Center
900 SW 16th Street, Suite 100

Renton, WA 98057

Online: <cancercenter.com/seattle-clinic.cfm>

Phone: 800-931-9299

Southwestern Regional Medical Center

Cancer Treatment & Wellness Center

10109 East 79th Street (81st Street & Highway 169)

Tulsa, OK 74133

Online: <cancercenter.com/southwestern-hospital.cfm>

Phone: 918-286-5000

Western Regional Medical Center

Cancer Treatment & Wellness Center

14200 W. Fillmore Street

Goodyear, Arizona 85338

Online: <cancercenter.com/western-hospital.cfm>

Phone: 623-207-3000

Southeastern Regional Medical Center

Cancer Treatment & Wellness Center Georgia to open August 2012

Online: <cancercenter.com/cancer-hospitals/southeatern-project.cfm

**An apple a day may keep the doctor away,
but cole family vegetables keep cancer at bay.**

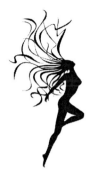

Chapter Thirty-Seven
Molecular Medicine Doctors
Medical Doctors Who Treat the Entire Body Holistically

Stay close to nature and its eternal laws will protect you.

… Max Gerson, MD (1881—1959)
German-born cancer researcher/MD

*D*id you know that the World Health Organization (WHO) in its report "The World Health Report 2000" states:

> *The U.S. health system spends a higher portion of its gross domestic product than any other country but ranks 37 out of 191 countries according to its performance,* *the report finds. The United Kingdom, which spends just six percent of GDP on health services, ranks 18th.* ***Several small countries – San Marino, Andorra, Malta and Singapore are rated close behind second-placed Italy.***
> [CJF emphasis added]

What most allopathic conventional medicine practitioners don't realize is that any disease in the body *affects the entire body*, not just a specific organ, tissue, or pathway the disease is centered in, such as diabetes or heart disease. Supporting all biochemical systems—the whole body and its return to health—is how the term holistic medicine evolved.

However, recently the term holistic is being replaced with *molecular medicine*. The reason is because physicians who utilize nutrients in their treatments are working at molecular levels to provide *nutritional cellular/molecular* support which, in turn, activates human biochemistry to work as it was designed to but doesn't due to disease, trauma, chemical toxicity, genetics, vaccine adverse reactions—either immediate or long-term—infection, inflammation, or psychosomatic-induced issues, such as post traumatic stress disorder (PTSD).

Molecular medicine physicians, therefore, really don't treat cancer *per se*; they treat the patient as a whole entity building up and revitalizing the immune system; whereas, conventional allopathic physicians really do treat cancer with surgery-radiation-chemotherapy, most of which are toxic and further impair the immune system.

You never will find allopathic cancer treatments in holistic physicians offices because they really don't treat cancer: *They guide the entire body into a state of health and wellness—homeostasis,* since the body inherently is designed to heal itself, and has been doing that for thousands of years before allopathic medicine, the chemo-pharmaceutical industry, and federal health agencies like the CDC and FDA came on the scene within the last hundred years or so—which, by the way, have created a monopoly in healthcare and cancer treatments, in particular.

One could say there is a huge philosophical divide between what conventional cancer treatment physicians view as holistic 'quackery' and what the allopathic monopoly establishment, in fact, provides as approved and effective cancer treatments. Why do cancer patients get "chemo brain," lose their hair, suffer radiation burns, etc.? *MedlinePlus* published online Robert Preidt's article "Breast Cancer Treatment Side Effects May Last for Years" April 11, 2012 [<nlm.nih.gov/medlineplus/news/fullstory_123977.html>] wherein he reported an Australian study that

> *Researchers looked at 287 Australian breast cancer patients and found that more than 60 percent of them had at least one treatment-related complication up to six years after their diagnosis, and 30 percent had at least two complications.*

Preidt went on to quote Kathryn Schmitz, associate professor of biostatistics and epidemiology at the University of Pennsylvania, as saying,

> *"We can no longer pretend that the side effects of breast cancer treatment end after patients finish active treatment. The scope of these complications is shocking and upsetting, but a ready solution for many of them already exists in rehabilitative exercise,"* [119]

Allopaths (oncologists, radiologist, cancer surgeons, etc.) treat cancer, whereas *molecular medicine physicians* would never 'go there' with chemotherapy treatments that basically are anathema to their holistic practice. In a sense, molecular medicine physicians are '*body re-builders*'. Instead of tearing down the body's immune system with radiation and toxic chemicals, molecular medicine physicians rebuild it with diet, nutrition, supplements, and *nutraceuticals*. Those modalities work to return the body to its natural healthy functioning capability to deal with and repair unhealthy issues going on at cellular or molecular levels.

Following is a list of physicians who practice molecular medicine. *They treat the entire body.* However, there are clinics in other countries that say they treat cancer. There's a listing of those facilities at the end of this chapter.

USA-Based Molecular Medicine Physicians

Keith I Block, MD
Block Center for Integrative Cancer Care
1800 Sherman Avenue, Suite 515
Evanston, IL 60201
Phone: 847-492-3040
Website: <blockmed.com>

Jeanne Drisko, MD
Program in Integrative Medicine
3901 Rainbow Blvd., Mail Stop 2028
Kansas City, MO 66160
Phone: 913-588-6208
Email: <jdrisko@kume.edu>
Website:

James W Forsythe, MD, HMD
Century Wellness Clinic
521 Hammill Lane
Reno, Nevada 89511
Phone: 775-837-0707

Elson Haas, MD
Preventive Medical Ctr of Marin
25 Mitchell Blvd., Suite 8
San Rafael, CA 95903

Phone: 415-472-2343
Email: lora_pmc2000@hotmail.com
Website: <elsonhaas.com>

Michael Schachter, MD
Schachter Complementary Medicine
Two Executive Blvd., Suite 202
Suffern, NY 10901
Phone: 845-368-4700
Website: <mbschachter.com>

Robert Jay Rowen, MD

PO Box 817
Santa Rosa, CA 95402
Phone: 707-578-7787
Email: terrisu@sonic.net

Toll free: 877-789-0707
Website: <centurywellness.
com>

Michael Galitzer, MD
American Health Institute

12381 Wilshire Blvd., Suite
102
Los Angeles, CA 90025
Toll free: 800-392-2623
Website: <ahealth.com>

Naima Abdel-Ghany, MD
Amal Medical Clinic

340 West 23rd Street, Suite K

Panama City, FL 32405
Phone: 850-872-8122

Website: <bioimmune.com>

Garry Gordon, MD

Gordon Research Institute
600 N. Beeline Highway,
Suite B
Payson, AZ 85541
Phone: 928-472-4263

Website: <doctorrowen.
com>

Charles Simone, MD
Simone Protective Cancer
Center
123 Franklin Corner Road

Lawrenceville, NJ 08648
Phone: 609-896-2646
Website: <drsimone.com>

Julian Whitaker, MD
Whitaker Wellness Institute
Medical
4321 Birch St-NewportBch
CA92660
Toll free: 800-488-1500
Email: <info@witakerwell-
ness.com>

Website: <whitakerwellness.
com>

**Nicholas J Gonzalez, MD,
PC**
Linda L Isaacs, MD
36A East 36th Street, Suite
204
New York, NY 10016
Phone: 212-213-3337

Website: <gordonresearch.com>

Website: <drgonzalez.com/index>

USA Physician Who Specializes in and Treats Cancer

Stanislaw Burzynski, MD, PhD
Burzynski Clinic
9432 Old Katy Road, Suite 200
Houston, TX 77055
Phone: 713-335-5697
Email: <info@burzynskiclinic.com>
Website: <burzynskiclinic.com/drb.htm>

Note: Dr Burzynski's cancer treatments have been documented as valid by investigators from the National Cancer Institute when, in 1992, National Cancer Institute investigators examined medical records from seven terminally ill cancer patients. Their conclusion was that Dr Burzynski's treatments caused complete and/or partial remission of brain cancer in every case. MG Hawkins and MA Friedman reported on that investigation in a paper published in the *Journal of the National Cancer Institute*, 1992; 84: 22, 1701.

USA Clinics

The Gerson Institute

P.O. Box 161358, San Diego, CA 92176

(888) 443-7766 (619) 685-5353

Email: info@gerson.org

Website:

For an informative 8-minute interview with Charlotte Gerson, the late Dr Gerson's daughter, regarding her father's work she has continued with cancer patients, please watch <renegadehealth.com/gersontapes/special/>.

Here's a comprehensive website listing clinics and other resources

<cancertutor.com/Other/Clinics.html>

Foreign Clinics

Note: This information is offered as a resource only with no recommendations nor endorsements of any kind.

Please make certain to check out all details regarding payment, and *if* there is any health insurance coverage or reimbursement from your healthcare insurance company in the USA *before* making any decisions.

European cancer clinics information EuroMed Foundation Website:

European cancer treatment centers in

Austria, Germany, Hungary, Poland, United Kingdom, and Turkey

Website: <health-tourism.com/cancer-treatment/europe-3/>

German cancer clinics guide: ***German Cancer Breakthrough***

Website:

German cancer clinics: **Veramedica Institute**

Website:

IAT (Immune Augmentation Therapy) Cancer Treatment

Freeport, Bahamas

Website: <immunemedicine.com>

Mexico: Hospital Saint Marc, Tijuana, Mexico

USA phone number: 619-241-5853

This book's author met and talked with Dr Julian Mejia, MD, who uses holistic cancer treatments at Hospital Saint Marc, Mexico. I also interviewed a breast cancer patient survivor cured by following cancer protocols there. Her story appears in Chapter 38.

Mexico Resource for **five cancer clinics**

Website: <mexicancancerclinics.com>

South Africa *multi-disciplinary treatment clinic*

Mayo Clinic of South Africa / Life Extension Institute of South Africa

Website: <mayoclinic.co.za/life_extension_institute.htm>

Turkey Johns Hopkins-affiliated CyberKnife Treatment

Website: <medicaltourismco.com/oncology/cyberknife-cancer-radiotherapy-oversease.php>

If you don't succeed at first, try, try, and try again.

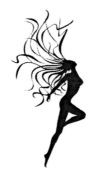

Chapter Thirty-Eight
Holistic Breast Cancer Treatments
Hospital Saint Marc (Mexico)
Julian Mejia, MD

Healing is a matter of time, but it is
sometimes also a matter of opportunity.

… Hippocrates (c.460 BCE—370 BCE)

The use of alternative therapies is growing as a result of more people looking for a natural approach to cancer. In fact, there are many alternative cancer options that have proven to be more effective than the conventional model.

As a physician treating cancer and other degenerative diseases, I use a multi-disciplinary approach of alternative/holistic therapies to support the patient. Cancer is addressed as a whole body disease. At our hospital metabolic therapies are based on the work of Dr Harold Manner and include laetrile, vitamin C, DMSO, and pancreatic enzymes. Other therapies are added to this protocol that are non-toxic or have minimum side effects.

I.D.E.A.S. is a step-by-step approach that individuals can implement in dealing with cancer or other degenerative diseases.

"I" is for the Immune System. The support of the immune system is a common denominator in all alternative therapies. The immune system controls the defense function of the body and depending on its strength, it can help prevent the disease process. There are many factors that affect immune function.

"D" is for Diet and Detoxification. It is well known that "we are what we eat." In the early years of alternative therapies, few believed that vegetarian diets, reduction in the consumption of red meat, and even the use of vitamins were helpful in reducing the risk of disease. Today, alternative and even some conventional studies show that diet and supplements are needed in the prevention and treatment of immune related diseases. A good, "clean" diet improves the elimination of waste and allows the intestinal tract to easily absorb nutrients.

Detoxification begins with an elimination of factors that may affect our health, as well as cleaning the physical body in different ways. Oriental medicine has many herbs and plants that accelerate liver detoxification. Coffee enemas are used as a liver and bile flush. Chelation, which means "pull out," is used to eliminate heavy metals, cholesterol, and other toxins from our blood stream.

"E" is for Enhancement. The basic premise of improving or enhancing the immune system is another step in the process.

This increase in the immune function can be accomplished by dietary products (vitamin C, turmeric, grape seed extract…), administration of autogenous vaccines extracted from a patient's own urine (polypeptides, interferon, interleukins…) or external products (Pind-A-Vi, Eurixor-Mistletoe, New Castle Virus, Transfer Factor-AF2…). This approach accelerates the production of the immune system elements to prevent cancer cell growth or to attack degenerative cancer cell growth, as well as eliminating dead cancer cells via macrophages.

"A" is for Approach. Alternative and metabolic therapies described by Dr Harold Manner in the early 1970s rebalance the entire body system through the use of natural and nutritional approaches. These approaches make the body stronger and more capable of eliciting a better immune response. In addition to the immune stimulating agents previously discussed, Major Autohem Therapy (IV Ozone) is used to increase oxygenation in the blood stream. Malignant cells cannot survive high concentrations of oxygen. Another therapy, intravenous cesium chloride (CsCl), has been used in the last fifteen years. This approach elevates the pH of the body to levels where cancer cells cannot survive.

"S" is for Supplements and Stress. Supplements are a fundamental part of cancer treatment. Most patients do not properly absorb or metabolize their nutrients. Therefore it is essential to have a proper supplement program. Vitamins (A, C, D, E), minerals, and other nutrients are part of the alternative protocol. An important factor in the treatment of breast and prostate cancer is the proper balancing of hormones.

Many studies confirm that stress creates disease and shortens our lives. It decreases the function of the immune system. There are simple changes that can be made to help reduce the stress level. Exercise is a valuable tool in controlling stress. It helps to pump blood and improves oxygenation of the body. It improves sleep and appetite. Health needs to be a priority. Therefore, anything negative or toxic (thoughts, relationships, habits...) should be eliminated.

The alternative/holistic protocol is a two-part process. Initially patients are seen as an inpatient or outpatient at the facility in Mexico. After the 14-21 day program, patients are given a protocol to follow after returning home. Patients remain in contact with the managing physician via phone/email consultations. Booster programs are determined on an individual basis.

Cancer is not about treating the tumor but in finding ways to support the immune function within the body. Ultimately, it is the immune system that attacks the cancer. Alternative/holistic therapies understand and utilize this basic premise.

Dr Julian Mejia, MD

Dr Mejia has treated patients from around the globe at clinics in Mexico. Currently he is attending patients at Saint Marc Hospital in Tijuana, Mexico, where Lisa Weir, a breast cancer patient, went for treatment. Below is Mrs Weir's essay about her treatments and recovery using Dr Mejia's protocols. Lisa is a ten-year breast cancer survivor.

Lisa Weir, Ten-Year Breast Cancer Survivor
Lisa's Story About Holistic Breast Cancer Treatment

Ten years have passed and only recently have I been willing to tell my story. I know the only way to get out the word about alternative or holistic cancer treatments is to talk about our successes. The conventional (allopathic) medical community is not interested in questioning the conventional treatment model. So, that's our job. We need to be catalysts in this venture and our own patient advocates for our healthcare. Education is the first step.

At my initial diagnosis of breast cancer, I was in shock. I thought that there was a stereotypical breast cancer patient, i.e., stress, unhealthy relationships, poor eating habits. Well, that wasn't me, was it? Not only was I wrong; I was embarrassed to even admit I was so ignorant. Cancer is not so simple.

Late in 2001, I was diagnosed with *stage 2 invasive ductal carcinoma.* I knew immediately that I was choosing alternative aka holistic treatment options to fight this battle. Perhaps you need to know a little about my family to understand my motivation and desire to use alternative methods.

Seven years prior, I lost my sister to breast cancer at the age of thirty-six. Although we grew up in a family of chiropractors, we had very little knowledge about alternative/ holistic cancer treatments. Kathy, my sister, was only 31 when she was diagnosed. I did all of her research for her health decisions and was excited to think that we had two comprehensive cancer centers in our area. "Great," I thought. "She will get excellent, state of the art medical care." She did it all too—surgery, chemotherapy, and radiation. But unfortunately, the cancer came back just months after completing the conventional protocol. And of course, there was nothing more "they" could do.

At that same time, my youngest sister, Karen, was in chiropractic school. She knew a woman whose mom was treated in Mexico. Back then there was no Internet. The only way to get information on alternative/holistic treatment was by word of mouth. Very few books were written on the subject, including books dealing specifically with breast cancer protocols from a patient's point of view.

When Karen called me to tell me about this clinic in Mexico, my exact words were, *"I am not taking our sister to a clinic in a third world country that probably uses dirty needles."* Doesn't the United States have the best healthcare in the world, I thought? Twenty years later I am confessing just how shortsighted, uneducated, and totally wrong I was.

Long story short, we did just that. When the medical community told us there was nothing more to be done for her, "Get your affairs in order," we headed south to Mexico. And that is where I met Dr Julian Mejia, a *licensed* Medical Doctor.

Dr Julian Mejia was clinical director at Manner Clinic in Tijuana, Mexico. Dr Harold Manner, founder of the clinic, was from Northwestern University in Illinois. He was one of the early, prominent practitioners of laetrile (B17), incorporating it into the "Manner Cocktail," which included an intravenous solution of Vitamin C, DMSO (dimethyl sulfoxide), and laetrile. Kathy used this alternative approach for her advanced stage breast cancer and lived another 3 ½ years with quality added to her life, after having been told, in essence, 'get ready to die' years earlier by cancer specialists in the USA.

Fast forward to 2001, and I am faced with a premenopausal breast cancer diagnosis. My first call was to Dr Mejia at Hospital St Marc in Playas, Mexico. I decided to have surgery first in order to reduce my tumor burden. Less than three weeks after a mastectomy, I was on my way to Mexico.

Dr Mejia uses the "Manner Cocktail," supplementation, detoxification, diet, and education to assist the patient in healing. You can choose to be an outpatient, staying at a local hotel, or an inpatient at the hospital. I previously had been to Mexico with my sister and was familiar with the area, so I chose to be an outpatient. My initial stay was approximately two weeks with a follow up visit scheduled six months later. Since that time, I have been back to St Marc periodically to boost my immune system and to check in with Dr Mejia.

My approach to cancer has been a multi-disciplinary approach. I believe that healing the body physically from cancer is not about finding the "silver bullet" but in designing a protocol that fits your needs. You are the captain of your team of health care professionals. You have the final say. You need to be educated and must question everything.

In addition to my therapies at St Marc with Dr Mejia, I also followed the Kelley Metabolic Program. This protocol was based on the use of pancreatic enzymes, proper supplementation, coffee enemas, and a nutritional program based on my metabolic type. I have also used Essiac tea, herbal remedies, *Iscador,* juicing, and the proper balancing of hormones estrogen and progesterone as prescribed.

Detoxification was an important aspect to my healing. On a daily basis my body was bombarded by toxins through my diet, my environment, plus my personal care and cleaning products. When I was a young child growing up in the sixties, a truck sprayed for mosquitoes in our neighborhood. My late sister Kathy and I would ride our bikes in the white cloud of DDE, the sweet smelling chemical linked to breast cancer. My brother, also a chiropractor, suggested a detox program through Dr Conrad Maulfair, a holistic physician in our region. The program is based on the work of L Ron Hubbard in his book *Clear Mind, Clear Body.*

As part of the protocol, Dr Maulfair suggested a fat biopsy to see whether I had DDE stored in my fat tissue. The results showed unbelievably high levels of DDE and DDT. Six months after completing the program, I had a follow up fat biopsy and the levels were dramatically reduced.

Throughout my healing, with every therapy, every lifestyle change, every diagnostic test, every book I read, every prayer I prayed, I faithfully saw my chiropractor. I know, no matter what I did, in order to receive the maximum benefit, I had to make sure that my nervous system was working at 100 percent efficiency without any interference in order to keep maximum electromagnetic energies flowing throughout my body.

I also understand that cancer is not just a physical disease. It is not just about treating the tumor, which is only a symptom of cancer. The immune system needs to be supported. Healing must take place on all levels: spiritually, psychologically, emotionally as well as physically.

Cancer healing has been a process for me. I have grown in my ability to care for myself. My priorities have shifted. I now say "no" more frequently. I manage my career, my family relationships, and social obligations more carefully. I am disciplined about meditation and my quiet time. I surround myself with positive people in a supportive environment. Stress will always be a part of my life but I am learning to handle the stressors more effectively.

In the beginning, every day I made a commitment to get well. On those especially hard days, I just persevered. Can I do this for just today? When I looked at the total picture, it was too overwhelming, but when I looked at the day, or even the next hour, I knew I could continue on always, always with the end result in mind. I was going to survive. And so I have; it's ten wonderful years and still counting.

Lisa Weir

The most important thing one can do is believe.

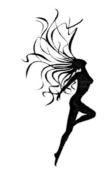

Chapter Thirty-Nine
Acupuncture

In short, it [acupuncture] provides maximum benefits without the dangerous side effects associated with many of the approaches of conventional medicine.

… William Michael Cargile, BS, DC, FIACA
Chairman of Research
American Association of Acupuncture and Oriental Medicine

*A*cupuncture is dubbed as an alternative healthcare treatment—or alternative medicine, which to my way of thinking is way out in left field. Now why would I make such an apparent mis-statement? Well, to begin with, acupuncture has been a part of Traditional Chinese Medicine (TCM) for millennia. How is *that* an alternative?

Perhaps one could claim that allopathic medicine—the pharmaceutical-industry-led healthcare system (20th century CE) that evolved into a predatory healthcare force—is *the* alternative—and for several reasons. One reason, for example, is something called *iatrogenic illness*, which results either from allopathic treatment, prescription drugs, vaccines, or nuclear medicine. It is estimated that in the United States alone, there are 225,000 *deaths annually* caused by iatrogenesis [120], i.e., caused by medical treatment or advice. Sad as it for me to say, conventional cancer treatment falls within that category. But look what Dr Grisanti also said in his article "Iatrogenic Disease: The 3rd Most Fatal Disease in the USA,"

> *The poor performance of the U.S. was recently confirmed by a World Health Organization study which used different data and ranked the United States as 15th among 25 industrialized countries.* [120] [CJF emphasis added]
>
> *It has been known that drugs are the fourth leading cause of death in the U.S.* [120]

Allopathic oncology treatments border on torturous in scope, as many people who have gone through them say. That's why they opt out for holistic treatment in many instances. But here's what I can't seem to grasp. Conventional medicine claims it has the 'gold standard' of treatment for cancer, yet it loses patients either to death or holistic medical practices. Furthermore, allopathic oncology medicine will fault and denounce any healing approach as quackery and unscientific other than its ionizing-radiation-chemotherapy-based protocols. Well, from where I come, when allopathy has been around as long as acupuncture has, healing people as effectively as it has, then allopathy can start to blow its horn. Until then, I think it ought to be a little more humble and take some pointers from modalities like acupuncture, an over 4,000 year old proven modality. Nothing would last four thousand years if it didn't work. Isn't that proof?

Acupuncture is based in the principle of energy streams within the body, or *chi,* also known as *qi.* Since the human body functions via electrical impulses, which mainly is understood by most folks as activity within the brain—neurons and synapses—electrical energy coming out of the brain flows throughout the body via meridians that can become blocked or stagnant. Chinese acupuncturists ages ago knew and practiced what in recent years has become known as "energy medicine." Chiropractic also is based on similar energy principles with subluxations being defined as the impediment to energy flow.

Backing up a little, Traditional Chinese Medicine can be traced back as far as the legendary reign of *Huangdi,* The Yellow Emperor, over four thousand years ago. With such a *pedigree* how can acupuncture be called an 'alternative'?

The chart below shows the directional flow of energy meridians and the flow of chi, which is correlated with the concept of yin and yang. Since energy flows to all organs that have their designated and respective yin or yang status under TCM, illness, pain, etc. happen when a yin organ or pathway becomes yang, or vice versa. Inserting acupuncture needles into proper meridians opens or unblocks them, corrects the flow of chi, and promotes healing due to electrical impulses needed for proper function. A similar concept or analogy could be compared with a blocked sewer line or a short circuit in an electrical appliance.

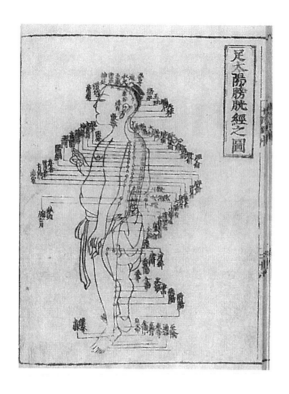

Acupuncture chart from Hua Shou
(fl. 1340s, Ming Dynasty).

This image from Shi si jing fa hui (Expression of the Fourteen Meridians). (Tokyo: Suharaya Heisuke kanko, Kyoho gan 1716). Courtesy of Wikipedia's Creative Commons Attribution Share Alike License

An acupuncturist makes a diagnosis after a lengthy review of a person's oral and written health history, visual examination of the tongue and skin, plus a TCM-technique of examining the pulse for rhythm, strength, and volume that is counter to western medicine's pulse-taking, which is just a number count.

Stainless steel, sterile, one-time-use needles are inserted in as many as two or three dozen acupoints all over the body from head to toe—literally to the tip of the big toe sometimes, depending upon what the acupuncturist decides after examination.

I can assure you that after having five days in a row of acupuncture sessions, I did not feel or leak like a sieve, nor did I experience any discomfort upon the insertion of those very thin needles. Sometimes as soon as the needle was inserted, I felt what I would call a relief or openess in my body.

As with any type of bodily treatment, there can be an adverse reaction, which is extremely low for acupuncture. Thankfully, and to its credit, acupuncture often relieves allopathic health practice mistakes. For those who doubt the capabilities for which acupuncture can be used medically, may I suggest reading a rather detailed analysis of what researchers, medical doctors, and others have reported on the website *Science-Based Medicine* at <sciencebasedmedicine.org/index.php/acupuncture-anesthesia-a-proclamation-of-chairman-mao-part-i/>. Personally, my first recommendation would be to acquaint yourself with as much information as possible about acupuncture, and then seek out a licensed professional who has been trained in traditional acupuncture, if you want to avail yourself of its health-generating practices, which can include certain herbs, nutritional supplements, and other techniques like moxibustion and cupping, *IF* and when you deem it appropriate for you. Interestingly, some health insurance companies will cover acupuncture when you have a medical doctor's prescription for treatment. Again, you will have to do your homework with your health insurance company and doctor.

I say don't knock it until you've tried it.

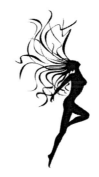

Chapter Forty
Chiropractic and Cancer Management
Leo McCormick, DC

Do not forget that chiropractors did not treat diseases.
They adjust causes, whether acquired, spontaneous,
or the result of accident.

… DD Palmer (1845—1913)
Founder of chiropractic

Just the word chiropractor sparks debate. Mention chiropractic with cancer treatment and you are stretching the sensibilities of most people. Well, are you really? If you just consider the body and how it functions, you will see that chiropractic is as sensible as eating healthful, natural foods, and breathing clean fresh air.

The human body is the most advanced 'machine' ever developed to date.

Generally, most people have a basic knowledge of how to keep a body operating. I tell my patients, "Just ask your grandma and she'll tell you what to do: Eat three squares, drink lots of water, work hard, and get sleep." Follow these golden rules and the human machine usually will run well. Sounds good, but it does not always work consistently. Disease can set in no matter how well you follow those golden rules. That is where a doctor of chiropractic, the chiropractor, is able to help. A chiropractor's expertise is in the manipulation of the spine and structures of the body to stimulate the nervous system. A healthy body must include a healthy nervous system.

Chiropractors are specialists in that aspect of health and certainly deserve mention in the management of any health issues, including preventive measures and the management of cancer, including breast cancer.

Largely misunderstood due to allopathic medical suppression and poor information to the public over the years, chiropractic has seen a resurgence in the past decade, is the largest *natural healing* profession, and the fastest growing segment of the health care field.

The basic premise behind chiropractic is that a healthy spine represents a healthy you. This is true because it is well researched and a known fact that the nervous system is the master system of the body. Without it, nothing in the body functions well or functions at all. Humans are constantly in a state of breakdown and repair in the body. When that repair process is faster than the breakdown, we call that health. When the breakdown is faster than the repair, we call that sickness or disease.

All repair processes are governed and controlled through the nervous system. Thus, if the nervous system is compromised in any way your body runs less efficiently, and that includes fighting off disease. The most common cause of nervous system stress and dysfunction is spinal tension caused by spinal misalignment and the resulting poor mechanics of the spine. That is called a **subluxation** by chiropractors. A variety of chiropractic techniques are employed to relieve the body of these health-robbing subluxations. All chiropractic techniques and approaches are effective; a patient just needs to find one that works for them to align neuro-physiological impulses.

The beginnings of chiropractic can be traced to 1895 and Dr Daniel Palmer of Davenport, Iowa. He surmised that the cause of Mr Harvey Lillard's deafness (Dr Palmer's janitor) was because Harvey strained his back when lifting. Upon examination Dr Palmer found a vertebra out of position, pushed it into place and Harvey's hearing was restored. From that basic story starts the amazing history of chiropractic. Little did Dr Palmer realize that stimulating the nervous system via an adjustment to the spine has been documented as far back as the time of the Egyptian pyramids. Nor did he realize that consistent nerve tension and pressure can cause disease in the body and that the restoration of this vital nerve energy can cause proper function to return to any diseased or dysfunctional organ.

This principle of nervous system health is vital for every person who is being treated for cancer. Chiropractic is good for every person's body. Why? Well the science behind it is very simple. In places where the spine has gone out of its normal optimal operating position resulting in subluxation, that nerve tract becomes irritated. That area then stops moving freely. The joints become fixated and toxins build up that encourage further dysfunction. That specific nerve track then will function less, react slower, and do the job of managing the health of the target organ or muscle in a far less optimal manner. Only a portion of that nerve is dedicated to pain sensation and transmission, so using pain as a guide, to function is limited at best. Most of the nerve is used for function. This includes the function of ALL the muscles, joints, and organs. Cut or sever a nerve to an organ, and you learn how quickly that organ becomes damaged and diseased. Putting pressure on that nerve from subluxation means we all ultimately get diseased and die even if it is slow and not readily observable.

Remember, our bodies are constantly breaking down and repairing, and when that breakdown occurs faster than the repair process, we are in a state of disease. At that point we begin experiencing visible symptoms and signs of disease. But we should ask when did the disease process start? Well, it occurs at the cellular level of that first subluxation. So does subluxation cause cancer? No. Your body constantly fights off cancer cells that are produced and subsequently are eliminated by your immune system. However, subluxation slows down the body's immune response mechanism to that cancer cell. Subluxation allows poor health to ultimately take hold of an otherwise healthy body.

People equate lack of pain or symptoms as an indicator of good health but *Dorland's Medical Dictionary's* definition of health is a state of complete physical, mental, and social well being, and not merely the absence of disease and infirmity.

Therefore, real health and its attainment is not just a decrease or elimination of pain or symptoms. Actually, the attainment of health is centered on a proper functioning of one's nervous system. Your local chiropractor is well equipped to take you to healthier realms previously not considered.

Chiropractic Breast Cancer Management

How does a chiropractor manage a person with cancer and other health issues? First and foremost, knowing the fact that the body functions and heals better with minimal spinal stress from subluxation, the chiropractor will do an examination to discover these areas of dysfunction. The chiropractor will physically examine the spine using palpation, muscle testing, orthopedic tests, and ranges of motion. The doctor may recommend various specific diagnostic testing consisting of radiographs (x-rays), blood work, surface EMG, MRI, ultrasound, and many others. Many patients have had this testing done prior to seeing a chiropractor and should take the results of those tests to the initial visit.

After evaluating the data, the chiropractor will design a treatment protocol for that specific patient to handle first any symptoms and then to restore proper function to the nervous system by the elimination of the subluxation. This treatment program may include stretches and exercises, as well as vitamins and supplements. Many chiropractors provide health classes to teach the specifics of stretches and good health habits.

Why seek chiropractic care when you are battling an illness or disease, especially breast cancer? Well simply stated, chiropractic care and the removal of the subluxation from the nervous system makes the body function better, improves the immune system, augments healing, and provides proper neuro-electrical impulses to diseased organs, including breast tissue. So whatever therapy you are using to restore your body to health, chiropractic will speed up the progress and make sure you are playing on an even field. Why let nervous system stress slow down the repair process? Chiropractic care gives your body the gift of health that emanates from the central nervous system.

Make your body a disease-fighting machine that God had intended it to be. Chiropractic care during breast cancer is important, especially today when most women work at computers for 8 hours a day, which often leads to subluxations of the thoracic area of the spine—that area that feeds nerve impulses to the female breasts. So, either as a breast cancer preventive measure or as an adjunct breast cancer treatment, chiropractic care ought to be included in your treatment protocol. You will be happy you made the decision.

Leo McCormick, DC

I repeat, don't knock it until you try it.

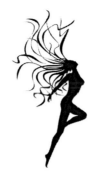

Chapter Forty-One
Dentistry, Is There a
Toxic Connection to Cancer?

Every tooth in a man's head is more valuable than a diamond.

... Miguel de Cervantes
***Don Quixote,* 1605**

*A*re there any connections with standard dentistry practices, e.g., silver amalgam (mercury) fillings, root canals, and fluoride to toxicity in the body or cancer?

Before I go further, my readers ought to know there are dentists who practice what is called holistic dentistry or *non-amalgam dentistry*, which means NO silver fillings that contain neurotoxic mercury.

The following web site <mercuryfreenow.com/freeservices/amalremov.html> is helpful in providing information locating mercury free dentists in the USA and safe amalgam removal. Then there's the six-minute *YouTube* video "Amalgam Stimulated With Soft Bristle Tooth Brush" <youtube.com/user/MercurySafe> that I encourage you to watch so that you can understand how dentistry and cancer may and can be connected.

Mercury is one of the most toxic substances in the world and yet it is placed into the human mouth over and over again from childhood on. In Chapter 19 *Toxic and Heavy Metals* of my last book, *Our Chemical Lives And The Hijacking Of Our DNA, A Probe Into What's Probably Making Us Sick,* I discuss mercury (Hg) with regard to dentistry.

What dental patients know as silver fillings really are an amalgamation of numerous components that shape up this way: One part is 50 percent mercury and the other 50 percent part is known as a *eutectic mixture* that consists of copper, tin, silver, and zinc.

All those metals are compounded into the amalgam that is placed into teeth that have been drilled to remove dental caries (decay). Now here's the unfortunate part about those amalgam fillings: They release mercury into the mouth and body, which causes toxicity within the body. Furthermore, old fillings that had been in the mouth for years and removed were assayed and found to contain only 24 to 26 percent mercury, when originally there was 50 percent mercury. Where did the mercury go? It went down the hatch every time you ate, drank food, brushed your teeth, or via fumes into the buccal/mouth cavity tissues that then traveled to other parts of the body. Mercury burdens the body with a heavy toxic load that contributes to many forms of disease, including cancer.

Cancer patients with amalgam fillings often have them removed and then go on a detox program to get out the mercury.

Removing mercury fillings is an art in itself, as there needs to be great protection taken with oral rubber dams placed in the mouth to prevent further absorption of the neurotoxic metal and fumes during removal.

The web site "Safe Removal of Amalgam Fillings" at <iaomt.org/aarticles/files/files288/Safe%20Removal1%20 of%20Amalgam%20Fillings.pdf> is extremely responsible in explaining the necessary precautions to be taken during the removal of mercury and amalgam fillings.

Before I leave amalgam fillings, I think you ought to know that several countries (Norway, Sweden, Denmark) have laws prohibiting amalgam fillings because mercury is a most dangerous environmental toxin.

Root Canals

The dental procedure known as root canal has become the gravy train of dentistry, I think. Just about everyone has a root canal in his or her mouth. I don't! Early in 2011, I was confronted with my first tooth problem that required a root canal at 72 years of age. Well, long story short, I told the dentist who had purchased the holistic practice where I'd been a patient since the 1980s—the former dentist retired—that it's either extraction or I leave and find another dentist. We had quite a conversation as to why I elected for the tooth to be extracted rather than have it 'saved'. How can you save a tooth when often infection is festering under the 'saved' tooth? That doesn't make much sense to me. One of the more predominant bacteria could be *Streptococcus*.

In the paper "The Effects of mechanical and chemical procedures on root canal surfaces" [121] the authors discuss "Residual bacterial infection in the root canal system after mechanical debridement" along with "*The average success rate of root canal treatment has been reported to be 74% with a range of 31—100%...*" [121] Furthermore, the chemicals used to kill the nerve in order to save the tooth, are—you got it—toxic, otherwise how could they kill the root? And often left inside your jaw and body thereby contributing to possible health problems.

There seems to be a coincidence of factors involved with root canals, and it is, most folks who contract cancer usually have a root canal in their mouth. Dr Hal Huggins, DDS, has done extensive research in this area and has written an interesting dissertation titled "Root Canals & Cancer" online at <whale.to/d/root2.html>. One of the dangers of root canals is immune dysfunction.

Once you understand the physiology of the underside of a root canal, I think, you then may understand why holistic cancer treatment includes extraction so that the infection can be cleaned out and the jaw tissue can heal. But then there still is the question of the toxic material that was used to kill the root. It still may be lodged in body tissue, which means a detoxification program ought to be undertaken to remove it.

The Other Tooth Fairytale: Fluoride

Fluoride is a protoplasmic poison and should not be used as a dental prophylactic, e.g., a dental treatment every six months, or in toothpaste for daily brushing of the teeth. Fluoride is an active ingredient in pesticides and rodenticides. It also is a base of some chemotherapy drugs to kill cancer cells. The web site <fluoridealert.org/health/> will tell you more about fluoride than you probably will want to know. Fluoride also is in municipal water systems, which is detrimental to everyone's health, especially cancer patients.

Laugh and the world laughs with you;
cry and, sadly, you cry alone.

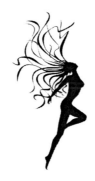

Chapter Forty-Two
Homeopathy and Cancer

Homeopathy cures a larger percentage of cases than any other method of treatment and is beyond doubt safer and more economical and most complete medical science.

**... Mahandas K Gandhi (1869—1948)
Political & ideological leader of India**

*U*pfront and straight out of the shoot, this is what I think you ought to know about homeopathy: The American Medical Association (AMA) was founded in the late 1840s to destroy homeopathy, which had a better cure record than other physicians who were bleeding their patients, often causing deaths.

Homeopathy is the healing practice of *like curing like* based upon the principles founded by Dr Samuel Hahnemann (1755-1843), a German physician who claimed medicine practiced during his time did as much harm—or more—than it did good. Hahnemann went on to invent homeopathy while experiencing an *aha* moment while translating *A Treatise on the Materia Medica* by William Cullen from English into German in 1790.

Dr Hahnemann's research included numerous trial and error procedures until he came up with succussion [systematic mixing via vigorous shaking], potentization [dilution and succussion process to make a certain potency], and subsequently, trituration [mixing or grinding substances with lactose] procedures for creating homeopathic remedies, as they are known, using various substances, which can be plants, minerals, and naturally-occurring products, e.g., animal bone, snake venom, etc.

To understand homeopathy, which can be considered as an adjunct to energy medicine, one has to get one's mind around the concept of potency. Homeopathics are made into potencies from 3X, 6X, 12X, 30C up to 50M to 100,000M, which are intricate in describing and to which I refer you to *Wikipedia*'s web site instead of my belaboring it here. Please see <en.wikipedia.org/wiki/Pontentization#The_theory_of_infinitesimals>.

Many physicians use homeopathy as part of their repertoire in practicing holistic medicine. Personally, I have used homeopathic remedies since the 1970s. As a child I can remember seeing a homeopathic physician. There's a great encyclopedia-like formulary for homeopath remedies titled *Homeopathic Materia Medica* that lists all homeopathic remedies, uses, etc., which has been updated since the first edition in 1811.

Over the ensuing years, additional information has been included due to the innovative updating of homeopathy by such luminaries as Dr Constatine Hering (known for Hering's

Law of Cure) plus numerous contributions from practitioners in Brazil, England, France, Germany, Italy, and Spain. Europeans are more inclined to seek out homeopathic treatments than Americans. However, when the AMA started going after homeopathy, there were numerous homeopathic medical schools—a dozen or more, if I remember correctly—in the USA, which the AMA got closed, unfortunately for medicine in the USA. Ever since, allopathic medicine, under the auspicies of the AMA, has become a turf-protective and preditory professional union in collusion with the pharmaceutical industry, which I think is responsible for a lot of the healthcare problems we have today—so sorry to have to be so candid.

How does homeopathy and cancer fit together? There are numerous remedies and potencies that can help a breast cancer patient rebuild or reinforce the immune system, cope with nausea, pain, etc. When first I discovered my problem, I immediately contacted my homeopathic MD and was given a specific immune enhancer for cancer. There are three remedies in homeopathy specifically for cancer. Your homeopathic physician can discuss them with you, as only he or she will know *which is the correct one for your constitution and special medical diagnosis.*

Those physicians who may be reading this book who are interested in finding out more about homeopathy and cancer, may I suggest this book, *A Homeopathic Approach to Cancer* by Dr AU Ramakrishnan, MD and Catherine R Coulter (For Professionals).

For healthcare consumers, I think *The Consumer's Guide to Homeopathy,* by Dana Ullman, MPH, will really help you understand the modality. If you are interested in finding a homeopathic MD/DO in your area, you may want to contact the National Center for Homeopathy in Washington, DC. Their phone number is (202) 223-6182.

Here's an innovative approach I found online where you can type into a computer Q&A format a question to ask a homeopathic physician [MD, DO, ND] that may help you decide what can be done for cancer using homeopathy in conjunction with other modalities. Or, you may use it to take a read on homeopathy to find out if it is a modality you would like to add to your treatments. Please visit <justanswer.com/sip/homeopathy?r=ppc>.

Seek and ye shall find.

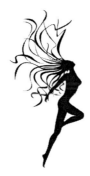

Chapter Forty-Three

Hyperbaric Medicine in Cancer Management
Hyperbaric Oxygen Therapy

Information is the oxygen of the modern age. It seeps through the walls topped by barbed wire, it wafts across the electrified borders.

… **Ronald Reagan (1911—2004)**
40ᵗʰ U.S. President

By the way: If you don't happen to know, President Reagan sought cancer treatment in 1985 from German medical doctor Hans Nieper. [122]

Although hyperbaric oxygen therapy is commonly used in treating decompression sickness, it is extremely effective in treating numerous other diseases, including cancer.

Before discussing hyperbaric oxygen in relation to cancer, here's a listing of other health conditions that can benefit from HBOT: Autism, ADD/ADHD, Cerebral Edema, Cerebral Palsy, Chrohn's Disease, Chronic Fatigue Syndrome, Fibromyalgia, Guillain Barré Syndrome, Immune System Dysfunction, Infection, Migraine Headache, Multiple

Sclerosis, Open Angle Glaucoma, Organic Brain Syndrome, Parkinson's Disease, Peripheral Neuropathy, ***Radiation Necrosis,*** Raynaud's Syndrome, Retinal Artery Occlusion, Rheumatoid Arthritis, Sports Injury, Stroke, Ulcerative Colitis.

Note ***Radiation Necrosis,*** which results from cancer radiation therapy, i.e., death of tissue from radiation treatment, can be helped by hyperbaric oxygen therapy (HBOT). Both the AMA and FDA approve HBOT for radiation injury. This website <florida-oxygen.com/html/radiation-necrosis> provides more information about it.

According to the *American Cancer Society's Find Support & Treatment* website,

> *Hyperbaric oxygen therapy involves the breathing of pure oxygen while in a sealed chamber that has been pressurized at 1-1/2 to 3 times normal atmospheric pressure. ...*
>
> *The U.S. Food and Drug Administration (FDA) has approved HBOT to treat more than a dozen health problems such as decompression sickness, carbon monoxide poisoning, gangrene, brain abscess, and injuries in which tissues are not getting enough oxygen. ...*
>
> *Research has shown HBOT can help when used as a mainstream treatment for the prevention and treatment of osteoradionecrosis, a term for delayed bone damage caused by radiation therapy. There is also some evidence suggesting HBOT may be helpful as an extra treatment for soft tissue injury caused by radiation. ...*

> *The FDA considers oxygen to be a drug, meaning it must be prescribed by a physician or licensed health care provider to treat illnesses or health conditions.* [123]

As justification for using HBOT (oxygen) in the treatment of radiation damage and cancer, I'm inclined to say HBOT makes a lot more sense than more chemotherapeutics since it's non-toxic and non-chemical, but a physician experienced in HBOT must administer it.

If HBOT may be considered as a cancer therapy per se, remember that it's scientifically known that cancer cells thrive in anaerobic conditions, i.e., low oxygen conditions, whereas when cancer cells receive or are exposed to extra oxygen, they literally suffocate and die. Cancer cells 'hate' oxygen and that's been established by medical science. However, Big Pharma can't make megabucks from HBOT—since it's not a patented pharmaceutical.

Something that I've heard cancer patients use to supply extra oxygen is 35% food grade hydrogen peroxide (H_2O_2), which has to be used with much care and strict guidelines, otherwise it can be dangerous. It also can be used to treat mold, wash vegetables, plus an array of other uses.

An excellent description of what oxygen does to cancer comes from the Sanoviv Medical Institute in Mexico website <sanoviv.com/health-concern/cancer/cancer-treatment.html?gclid=CN-Zn4z8oqwCFYHe4AodQSZM1w>.

Tumor hypoxia or lack of oxygen in tumor cells has proven to be a factor for poor prognosis in a cancer patient. Cancer cells cannot survive in an oxygenated environment. Oxygen therapy is another tool used to help fight cancer cells and reduce side effects from conventional cancer treatments. Many researchers think lack of oxygen in our cells is one of the primary causes of cancer. An impressive variety of new ways to introduce oxygen into the body is emerging. Flooding cells with oxygen may retard the growth of cancer cells or even help to return them to normal and maintain healthy cells at their normal functioning level.

To find more information about hyperbaric oxygen therapy, phone or email your request for a certified provider's name, clinic, or hyperbaric therapy center near you. Please remember to provide the city, address and state for a desired location.

Phone: 1-877-442-8721 or Email <info@ihausa.org>.

International Hyperbarics Association, Inc.

15810 East Gale Avenue #178, Hacienda Heights, California 91745 USA, 1-877-IHA-USA1

Website: <ihausa.org>

May I remind you that the American Cancer Society lists hyperbaric oxygen treatment on its web site <cancer.org/Treatment/ TratmentsandSideEffects/ComplementaryandAlternative Medicine/HerbsVitaminsandMinerals/hyperbaric-oxygen-therapy>.

I think that says something for the ACS in wanting to provide help for cancer patients harmed by radiation. If you visit their website you will see the page *Guidelines for Using Complementary and Alternative Methods* wherein ACS states,

Many insurance companies are starting to cover some of the more widely accepted complementary methods of treatment. Many major insurers, including Blue Cross and Medicare, cover one or more complementary methods of treatment. [123]

Under the ACS section *It's your call,* this appears:

The choice to use complementary or alternative methods is yours. You can use them more safely if...[123]

ACS lists numerous criteria, most involving allopathic medical doctors approval and/or input before using them. What can I say? At least the ACS has the good sense to make the suggestion and list complementary or holistic cancer treatments for which I congratulate and thank them.

I will put the wind beneath my wings and soar like an eagle to the heights.

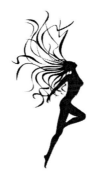

Chapter Forty-Four
Reiki, Does It Work?

*The most beautiful thing we can experience is the mystical.
It is the source of all true art and science.*

**... Albert Einstein (1879—1955)
Scientist/Educator**

$\mathcal{D}$r Einstein's quote ought to clue my readers that this chapter may not be about science, but about the mystical aspects of life, living, and the oneness of all. First and foremost, I must offer a caveat for those who may be concerned, the Roman Catholic Church in the United States in 2009 prohibited catholic hospitals and institutions from practicing Reiki. The reason given was that Reiki was not compatible with either the church's teaching or scientific evidence. That having been said, I will continue on with what I think may be helpful to your deciding *for yourself* if Reiki is something you may want to use in helping you cope with breast cancer.

A Japanese *Buddhist* monk, Mikao Usui, developed Reiki in 1922. Therein may be the problem insofar as *the battle of the ages,* i.e., ecumenism not crossing cultural barriers, in my opinion. Reiki is based upon spiritual principles of guiding or directing healing energy from the ultimate power of the universe, the energy that makes everything work, Creator God, the God Force, the Godhead, the Ultimate.

That's extremely esoteric, I agree. Nevertheless, if one believes in spirituality, then where is the problem? Is not the Creator the creator of all that is, was, and ever will be, including the Japanese? For me I cannot comprehend how invoking the ultimate in healing energy—the God Force—and sharing it with others through the placement of hands is outrageous or not compatible with Catholic doctrine. Don't Catholic priests do something similar in the Sacrament of the Sick with anointing the forehead (third eye or brow *chakra*) and the palms of both hands with blessed oil plus the over placement of the priest's hands in prayer to invoke healing—and to which I have availed myself often—as I truly believe that anyone who employs Creator God's healing energy and grace is something I want to have available to me in my quest for health and wellness.

Reiki works with the seven *chakras*—those energy centers within the human body that travel the spinal cord—to balance the flow of energy, or electro-magnetic impulses, throughout the body to encourage and assist in healing. That is something allopathic medicine—and I guess the RC church—cannot seem to accept: energy medicine, which is the medicine of the future, I think. However, the church and most spiritual persuasions accept the concept of a soul or one's spirit. Can't there be interaction by the spirit within a third dimensional frame known as the human body? Isn't that part of what the so-called 'junk' 90 percent of human DNA is about: encodements from Creator God?

Now, having given my short esoteric dissertation about energy medicine, which also includes homeopathy and chiropractic to a degree—both discredited by allopathy as 'quackery'—I will try to explain a little more in detail what Reiki is and does, keeping in mind that I'm not a Reiki master nor practitioner.

Basically, there are two forms of Reiki: *Traditional (Eastern)* as formulated by the Japanese monk Usui, and *Western,* a modernized version devised by Hawayo Takata in Hawaii during the late 1930s—the form that spread throughout the western world. It's a simplified version of the monk's more spiritual practices of Reiki, which concentrates on hand placements for energy flow and healing inducements.

The monk's form concentrated only on the head area energies, whereas the western version works on the entire body, especially areas of physical health anomalies or diseases, and the seven *chakras.* What are chakras, you may be asking? The word comes out of ancient Indian Hindu and Buddhist health practices that describe energy vortices within the human body that are comparable to modern medicine's endocrine system. For example: the brow chakra corresponds to the pituitary and pineal glands in the brain; the throat chakra, with the thyroid gland; the solar plexus chakra with the pancreas; the sacrum chakra, with the male and female hormonal and reproductive systems. Working from the head downward, the *chakras* are:

Seventh chakra, the Crown chakra, a couple inches above the head or crown

Sixth, the Brow or Third Eye chakra, in the center of the forehead between the eyes

Fifth, the Throat chakra, at the Adam's apple or thyroid area of the throat

Fourth, the Heart chakra, in the middle of the chest by the heart

Third, the Solar Plexus chakra, a hand width above the navel on the abdomen

Second, the Sacrum chakra, a hand width above the pubic bone on the abdomen

First, the Root or Base chakra, near the tailbone (coccyx) of the spine

Chakras are esoteric energy centers that correspond with the endocrine system, which pumps out hormones, those *body-made, life-processes-controlling chemicals* that keep glandular and cellular activity humming along in optimum health. When malfunctions occur due to deficiencies, accidents, pollution, etc., disease patterns set in.

Much oversimplified, there is a great deal more to disease than meets the allopathic paradigm of health and disease. It includes physical, emotional, mental, and spiritual aspects or input. The Institute of Noetic Sciences (IONS), founded by astronaut Edgar Mitchell as a result of his paranormal experiences in space, is doing an incredible job in trying to bridge the occult (hidden) with the scientific aspects of health. They do great work, in my opinion, and will be recognized at some future date for the amazing contributions they have made to the body-mind connection in health and healing.

Reiki is a discipline that works with receiving, transferring, and moving healing energy around a body. It can be applied to humans or animals, i.e., your pet cat, dog, horse, etc. *I think* it may work with energy received from numerous life-giving sources such as Creator God, and other energy forms such as the sun, air, food, emotions, intellectual stimuli, and believe it or not, extraterrestrial cosmic forces such as the moon and other cosmic bodies, i.e., planets. Everything is energy, including humans.

The moon's effect on Planet Earth's tides has been well known for ages. The full moon's effect on the human psyche is quite apparent—even accepted by science—since crime statistics reveal that during the full moon phase, more crimes occur.

There are energies in outer space, e.g., the Van Allen Belt, that affect various factors. Sunspots and cosmic storms send energy. Energy is all around us. We cannot deny it. It's what we truly are when we get down to it. The proof for my saying that is there's an energy that makes us alive, eventually departs or transitions, and our bodies are physically dead. The energy that kept us alive transformed into another dimension, which some call the hereafter, heaven—even hell for those who believe in it. Basically we deal with positive and negative energy all the while we are alive. So, why not concentrate on moving positive Creator-God given life energy to use, enjoy, and help others. *That's what Reiki is all about,* in my opinion.

Reiki practitioners go through training and can earn three areas of expertise:

First Degree: Elementary or Entry Teachings
Second Degree: Inner Teachings
Third Degree: Master

All degrees in western Reiki use hand placements, prayer, and relaxation techniques. There are neither curses nor diabolic rituals invoked or involved; it's just working with, sharing, and moving God's creative energy in the body.

Personally, I've enjoyed Reiki sessions over the years and have felt energy move.

So, what can Reiki do for breast cancer patients? According to the allopathic medical profession, not very much! The American Cancer Society has this to say, "*Available scientific evidence at this time does not support claims that Reiki can help treat cancer or any other illness. More study may help determine to what extent, if at all, it can improve a patient's sense of well being.*" However, I do know of an allopathic breast surgeon who is a Reiki master.

However, *The Wall Street Journal* of March 15, 2011 published the article "A Touch of Massage Therapy" wherein reporter Laura Johannes said,

> "*Cancer patients—due to the disease and to side effects of chemotherapy—often suffer from severe mental and physical fatigue, doctors say. Anxiety, nausea and pain are also*

common. In recent years, many cancer centers have been offering Reiki, a form of healing which originated in Japan in the early 1900s, according to scientific literature." [124]

But here's where I think the value of Reiki is to be found and which The *WSJ* article confirms:

"Reiki is often described as a treatment that helps life energy to flow in a patient—an explanation not generally accepted by scientists. Barrie Cassileth, chief of the Integrative Medicine Service at Memorial Sloan-Kettering Cancer Center in New York, calls the energy theory 'absurd' but says light-touch therapy can have a 'great relaxing effect' on cancer patients 'who are constantly poked, prodded and given needles'." [124]

Patients who constantly are poked, prodded, and given needles can relax with a caring, compassionate, and trained Reiki therapist who will facilitate relaxation, tension and stress release, plus move energy around the body, even though some may think that, that concept is truly absurd.

For healing to occur in any disease, and particularly with breast cancer, it's paramount that a woman can relax physically, emotionally, and mentally. The gentle touch of a Reiki practitioner, plus the soothing calmness that encompasses a session often becomes the highlight of a breast cancer patient's week. Please don't let others influence your ability to get well because of what they perceive as nonsense. Some people think what others try to mandate that cancer patients do, including not having choices in treatment, is totally outrageous. I happen to agree. I know; I experienced those pressures but did not give in.

Reiki, in my opinion, is a non-toxic, non-chemotherapeutic, and non-invasive therapy that can help a breast cancer patient cope with the daily grind and head trips one has to deal with while undergoing breast cancer treatments. Allopathic breast cancer treatments are not easy to take. It's easy for those who have not experienced breast cancer to say what they say, which I feel is totally insensitive. In my opinion, no one can understand what it's about until they have lived with it, and then it's a little too late with regard to retracting senseless insensitivities.

More and more breast cancer patients are finding their way onto Reiki therapists massage tables because they realize that for them, there *are* real benefits. Only you can decide what will work for you.

The International Center for Reiki Training has a web site listing practitioners in the USA, Puerto Rico, and Canada. If you would like to find a Reiki practitioner in your area, please visit their web site <reikimembership.com/MembershipListing. aspx>.

I'm full of energy, are you?

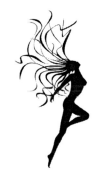

Chapter Forty-Five

Thermography

Philip Getson, DO, Board Certified Thermologist
and Liesha Getson, Board Certified Thermographic Technician

Trials can be rigged in a dozen ways, and it happens all the time.

... Marcia Angell, MD (1939—)
Former Editor-in-Chief, *New England Journal of Medicine*
Quoted from her book *The Truth About Drug Companies:*
How They Deceive Us and What to Do About It.

hermography, or infrared imaging, has its roots in the
military from the time of the Second World War. The
government equipped fighter planes with infrared imaging devices
that flew over missile silos. When the image showed excessive heat
it allowed the pilot to make the determination that these were
"active" missile silos that subsequently were targeted for destruc-
tion. "Cold" silos suggested lack of activity and were passed over.

Infrared imaging was not released for medical applications
until the 1950s. This date is significant as it predates mammography by over a decade.

With advances in technology and computer software packages, current infrared imaging devices allow for extremely sensitive determinations of various medical disorders including breast disease, neuromuscular disorders, thyroid, and dental issues. Current research is looking at other applications for infrared imaging as well.

I began performing thermography (the common name for infrared imaging) in the early 1980s. I felt even then that the technology lent itself to the determination of inflammatory conditions of the muscular and nervous system that would allow physicians yet another piece of information to assist them in the treatment of patients. Unfortunately, the insurance industry disagreed and refused to pay for the performance of this noninvasive diagnostic service. It should be noted that there were no needles, dyes, nor radiation thereby making it very different from the tests that were available at that time. (Remember that in the early 1980s there were no MRI machines.)

We continued to perform thermal imaging without auto accident liability insurance reimbursement and were very pleased with the results that we obtained. It allowed us to offer additional diagnostic criteria and recommendations for therapeutic intervention in a noninvasive fashion.

In an endeavor to foster recognition of this wonderful diagnostic tool (and to get paid as well), we filed a lawsuit against the two major auto insurance carriers in New Jersey, Allstate and State Farm, while suing the state health plan of New Jersey as well. This suit was filed in the 1980s and what followed was a seven-week trial in Camden County.

The results of that trial were such that the judge ruled in our favor and ordered payment of all outstanding bills for thermograms taken up to and inclusive of that point in time.

As expected, the insurers disagreed and filed an appeal, which was heard several years later by the Appellate Division court in New Jersey. They upheld the lower court's decision and ordered payment of outstanding bills.

Once again, the insurers disagreed filing an appeal that was heard by the Supreme Court of the State of New Jersey. For this appeal, both Allstate and State Farm brought in "house counsel" meaning that the lawyers who filed the necessary paperwork were the chief counsels of the parent insurance company in Illinois and Indiana.

It was interesting to note that one lawyer (mine) with his original law school briefcase and I presented in the Hall of Justice in Trenton, New Jersey, and were seated across the room from the lawyers representing the insurance industry in their expensive suits and even more expensive briefcases. I have often stated that the scene was reminiscent of Paul Newman's portrayal of a lawyer in the movie "The Verdict" in which one individual took on the legal establishment. The parallel continued, as the results were similar. The Supreme Court Justices ruled by a 5-0 vote in our favor therefore upholding both the lower court's decision and the appellate court's ratification of it.

Since that time, thermography or infrared imaging has been an integral part of my practice and recognized in the State of New Jersey as a valid diagnostic tool, in this case under the motor vehicle statute. There have since been innumerable instances of its recognition by workman's compensation carriers and other insurers.

Breast Thermography

In the last ten years the technology improved to the degree that breast thermography became an even more viable diagnostic tool than it had been previously. The performance of the test was far more cumbersome in the second half of the 20th century when the technology took a giant leap. We were able to move forward from the days of liquid nitrogen or contact thermography and use laptop computers and electricity based cameras that enabled us to perform very high-resolution infrared images of the breasts. By doing so we were able to study the breasts from a black and white perspective looking at vascular patterns and specific temperature gradients at and about the nipple as well as using multiple color palettes allowing us to identify regions of interest or concern in the breast comparing the heat pattern generated on one breast to its counterpart on the opposite or contralateral side.

Over the ensuing decade the technology has become even more sophisticated and refined allowing us to have a very high level of early screening for breast disease.

Physiologic versus Anatomic Tests

Thermography is a physiologic test as opposed to an anatomic one. The difference is quite simple. Anatomic tests look for distinct entities: tumors, cysts, and other kinds of masses that are identifiable in what we know as an anatomic sense. Thermography is a test that looks at the breast physiologically. The distinction is significant. Physiology is the determination of how things work while anatomy is the determination of how things look. Both are necessary in many instances to help render a diagnosis but it is important to note that in medicine (not just thermography) physiology <u>always</u> changes before anatomical entities are seen. Take, for example, a patient with pneumonia. The patient will be symptomatic with cough, fever, malaise, wheezing, etc. long before a chest x-ray will show the pneumonia. On the other end, the patient will improve and be symptom-free before the findings on the x-ray resolve.

This becomes not only interesting but important because some of the 800 or more peer-reviewed studies done worldwide describing thermal imaging have shown not only that thermography is the single best indicator for the earliest possible detection of breast disease but that, in some cases, these changes will occur seven to ten years before a mammogram will discern a lesion the size of a pencil eraser.

Consequential Results

The implication of this is tremendous. The American Cancer Society statistics show that one in eight women will ultimately be afflicted with breast cancer, a number that is twice as high as it was ten years ago. Largely this can be attributed to diet, environmental factors, toxins, etc. Therefore, a woman with an abnormal thermogram who does not have corresponding anatomic findings can now become proactive in her own health concerns. She can change her diet, eliminate toxic substances such as caffeine, sugar, alcohol, and tobacco and place herself on a regimen of vitamins and nutritional support products specifically directed to improving breast health. She can, in short, put herself in a position to improve her breast health and either minimize the risk of breast cancer or at least reduce the magnitude of the severity of the disorder. At the very least, she is going to be able to see changes of an anatomic nature at their earliest possible time as she monitors the physiologic abnormalities that thermal imaging offers.

Numerous experts in the field have described thermography as the first (and only) breast test that allows for early detection of breast abnormalities that can facilitate the earliest possible treatment and intervention.

We recommend breast screening as early as the late teens. With our estrogen-laden diets, females are developing breasts earlier and earlier and breast cancer is striking at an earlier and earlier age. As this is a diagnostic test without compression, radiation, injections, and in fact no contraindications, it is safe to do for teenagers. This allows for early monitoring of breast abnormalities that can ultimately lead to serious breast problems and even breast cancer. It allows for proactivity at an early age and becomes an ideal screening tool for that purpose.

It is well known in all fields of medicine that the earliest possible detection leads to the earliest and most successful treatment rates. It would therefore seem clear and evident that early breast screening will lead to better outcomes.

The American Cancer Society statistics show that one in eight women will ultimately be afflicted with breast cancer, a number that is twice as high as it was ten years ago. Largely this can be attributed to diet, environmental factors, toxins, etc. and so adjustments when possible in diet, the use of medication, exposure to noxious and potentially harmful chemicals, etc. would certainly minimize the incidence of breast cancer.

Other Thermographic Applications

Along the way we have determined that thermography is an excellent diagnostic tool for the evaluation of thyroid and dental disorders. Thyroid disease is poorly diagnosed by <u>conventional</u> diagnostic testing. Frequently the T3, T4, and TSH are normal in people who have clear-cut symptomatology of thyroid dysfunction. The physiologic nature of thermography allows us to determine that the thyroid is not functioning in a normal fashion and aids the clinician in moving forward with a program of thyroid related supplementation. Similarly, it has been suggested that dental infections are the only ones, which the body cannot heal in and of itself. We were able to localize inflammation, which may be associated with infection to quadrants of the mouth giving it a significant role in the earliest diagnosis and treatment of dental disorders.

Finally, the use of thermography in nerve related abnormalities such as, but not limited to, Complex Regional Pain Syndrome (Reflex Sympathetic Dystrophy), diabetic neuropathies, fibromyalgia, and certain types of other neuromuscular disorders has been noted in the medical literature as well. This is one of the only diagnostic tests that allows us to look at the physiologic functioning of the nervous system. This leads to a much greater understanding of physiologic neuropathic pain and has allowed for focused treatment.

Summary

The role of thermography has not yet been defined in its entirety. Current ongoing study worldwide will continue to find new applications for this diagnostic test. Because of its safety and lack of contraindication, it is suggested as a first-line-screening test in many disorders listed herein. It is, in my impression, the diagnostic tool of choice for the earliest possible detection of breast disease and the evaluation of patients with Complex Regional Pain Syndrome. It is an excellent assistive diagnostic tool in other neuropathic pain disorders as well as in thyroid and dental disease as well.

Philip Getson, DO and *Liesha Getson*

While waiting for Dr and Mrs Getson to write their contribution to the book, I wrote my 'two cents worth' of what I think about thermography, and it follows.

Before I get into discussing thermography, I must admit upfront that I am biased in favor of it and elected for thermography to be the diagnostic tool of choice for my situation. Why? Because I did not want to have ionizing radiation shot into my breasts and body, which is capable of inducing secondary cancers. Furthermore, I and numerous medical scientists and doctors consider thermography to be more accurate than mammograms, which notoriously have numerous false positive readings and diagnoses. Having divulged my personal feelings, now let's look at the science surrounding thermography from my perspective.

First, my readers ought to know that thermography is considered comparable to the devil by manufacturers of mammography equipment and their well-greased and funded lobbyists who influenced the U.S. Senate to support mammograms. In the summer of 1997 an organized effort swamped Congress to pass the *Mammography Quality Standards Act.* Delegate Eleanor Holmes Norton and Representative Nancy Johnson introduced a companion bill in the House of Representatives.

One can get an idea of what transpired from the abstract of the *JAMA* article "Preserving Scientific Debate and Patient Choice" by Drs Steven H Woolf and Robert S Lawrence that reported,

> *The National Institutes of Health (NIH) convened a consensus conference in January 1997 to examine new evidence on the effectiveness of mammographic screening for breast cancer in women ages 40 to 49 years. After reviewing the*

data and hearing testimony from experts and advocates, the panel concluded that the evidence did not support a universal recommendation for or against routine mammography in this age group.[1] *The panel advised each woman to decide with her physician, based on her personal values and risk factors, whether to have the test. Critics denounced this recommendation, accusing the panel of distorting the evidence and misleading the public.*[2] *News accounts emphasized the acrimony among health professionals and medical groups.*[3] *The US Senate passed a resolution repudiating the panel, demanded revised guidelines, and convened investigative hearings.*[4,5] [125]

During those investigative hearings much lobbying took place by those who had vested interests in the manufacture of mammogram machines and by others who believe mammograms are 'state of the art' diagnostics rather than potential cancer-inducing devices.

As always, there is politics in every issue and certainly the mammogram issue was a hot button item that did not lack for politicking. Considering that mammography is a $4 Billion a year industry in the United States alone, one can only imagine the pressure put on members of Congress to mandate mammograms yearly, even if they aren't effective at early detection.

Long story short, mammograms became part of the 'gold standard' of breast cancer diagnostics much to the unfortunate misdiagnoses of breast cancer. Why do I say that? Because mammograms usually are taken every year and yet women find out after years of having them, that all of a sudden, there's a tumor. How come mammograms didn't find it sooner? Thermography would have. How, you ask?

Thermography is capable of detecting abnormal blood flow into the tumor area in the breast(s) *years before* a tumor shows up on mammograms, and definitely before a female's routine breast self-examination finds a lump. Thermal imaging can detect changes at cellular level(s). Cancer cells produce heat that thermography photographs and coverts into a color spectrum graph of the breast(s). Furthermore, studies have shown that thermography can detect cancerous activity eight to ten years *before* other diagnostic tests, including mammography. Wouldn't you like to know sooner than later? Can you imagine what impact that has on the "early detection" advice? So why not use thermography on an annual basis knowing that it does not shoot ionizing, cancer-causing radiation into your body, and that it is so much more capable of finding problems years sooner. That, to my way of thinking, certainly is a no brainer.

Thermography detects thermal asymmetry from one side of the body to the other and has been approved by the U.S. Food and Drug Administration (FDA) since 1982 as an *adjunct* to mammography. So what's that all about? The politics of healthcare issues, like most issues the FDA is involved with. Probably not what works, but whose interests must be looked after, protected, and guaranteed. So what else is new?

In the mid 1960s I had several MDs fighting over the diagnosis that I had throat cancer, which I claimed I didn't because

I knew the way my throat was acting: the lump or swelling would go up and down. So, I finally demanded that I be evaluated by an Ear, Nose, and Throat specialist, and was fortunate to get the head of that division in a teaching hospital.

Long story short again, that ENT MD had a thermogram done on my neck, etc. and said, "No cancer, something else." I went through all kinds of tests to find out that I had infectious mononucleosis—mono, the "kissing disease" as they call it. The ENT doctor told me after being discharged from the hospital, that a young woman was in the same hospital as I with a similar diagnosis that I had—cancer of the throat—and surgeons operated, etc. She left the hospital in an undertaker's hearse. I was placed on a regimen of *Lincocin* (Lincomycin) and here I am almost fifty years later writing this book. So many years ago thermography was used not only to diagnose a condition for me, but as I feel, may have saved my life. So why shouldn't I trust it for my right breast problem?

Thermography is used to diagnose other conditions such as reflex sympathetic systrophy, thoracic outlet syndrome, peripheral neuropathies, fibromyalgia, peripheral vascular disease, thyroid assessment, temporomandibular joint dysfunction (TMJ), and dental infections that do not show up on X-ray.

Thermography is capable of monitoring nerve pathways that other physiologic tests can't.

Special cameras take photographs of the naked area under specific conditions, e.g., no cologne or other cosmetics, scented soaps, etc. before the test and the room temperature is kept at 68°F. For a breast thermogram, one must disrobe above the waist and sit in that cool room for the designated time prior to the photography session. Just think, you are posing for a center spread that probably will save your life. Then I was asked to hold an ice pack for several minutes and photos were taken again. That, basically, was the test: No hurtful squashing of my boobs between 50 to 60 pound weights that possibly could rupture the tumors, and most of all, no ionizing radiation.

As I write this chapter around Thanksgiving 2011, I feel that about 50 percent of the breast problem is gone. I plan on having another thermogram when I get the all clear from my managing holistic physician to make certain the camera captures the fact that I cured the tumors in my right breast using holistic therapies.

Where To Find Thermography Centers
Thermographic Diagnostic Imaging website <TDINJ.com>
The above provides information regarding thermography with photos, articles and breast healthy information
The American Academy of Thermology
Website <americanacademyofthermology.org>
ACCT Approved Thermography Clinics
Website: <thermologyonline.org/Breast/breast_thermography_clinics.htm>
The above lists ACCT-approved Thermography clinics in

- All states in the USA
- 18 foreign countries: Australia, Aruba, Canada, Caribbean, Cyprus, Denmark, Germany, Greece, India, Netherlands, New Zealand, Oman, Romania, South Africa, Spain, Sweden, Turkey, and United Kingdom.

This website discusses with photos, the Breast Screening Procedure

<thermologyonline.org/Breast/breast_thermography_procedure.htm>

This website includes Breast Screening Questions and Answers

<thermologyonline.org/Breast/breast_thermography_questions.htm>

Always remember when one door shuts, there's another door to open.

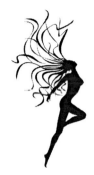

Chapter Forty-Six
Comments From Holistic Physicians

Health is the proper relationship between microcosm,
which is man, and the macrocosm, which is the universe.
Disease is a disruption of this relationship.

… Dr Yeshe Dhonden (1927—)
Physician to the Dalai Lama 1960 to 1980

Over the years I have had the greatest pleasure and blessing of being befriended by physicians, chiropractors, naturopaths, homeopaths, PhDs, holistic nurses, like-minded researchers, and holistic health practitioners of varied persuasions around the globe.

What strikes me as an oddity of sorts is that there is an overwhelming and ever-growing number of healthcare professionals who have gone through standard accredited academic and allopathic training only to realize after either personal experience or professional experience of not helping the sick and having no recourse to help them, that there is a faulty paradigm of sorts that just doesn't work when it comes to healing patients.

Their frustrations led to what is now called holistic/alternative/complementary healthcare. Conventional medicine calls it CAM—Complementary and Alternative Medicine. CAM practices and protocols that evolved have taken the best of many cultural and generational healing modalities, e.g., herbs, Chinese Traditional Medicine, Ayurvedic medicine, diet and nutrition—which are key, etc. and intertwined them with innovative technologies such as modern nutraceuticals and less invasive, non-toxic treatments while managing to practice the healing arts with greater satisfaction and healing prowess for their patients.

As I've admitted, I came to that conclusion when the conventional medical paradigm almost killed me a couple of times early in life. I came to the realization that there had to be something more reliable than the pharmaceuticals to which I had experienced numerous serious adverse reactions, almost to the point of killing me from adverse reactions. I am certain many physicians see the inadequacies of the allopathic system they are married into and from which they just can't leave either because of financial interests or peer pressure. That's why I admire and respect, with all my being, those healthcare professionals who have changed horses in midstream and now are providing non-toxic care, hope, and health.

I know what that feeling is like, as I experienced it for many years as a practicing *natural* nutritionist who would counsel medical doctors patients upon whom they had given up. The only modality I used was my educated knowledge of *natural* nutrition instructing my clients how to change diets and life-styles. *That's the real key to health.*

The successes I experienced with thousands of clients could fill a book. To this day I have clients who have found me via the Internet either emailing or telephoning to say thank you, and that they still live by the lessons I taught them. Not very long ago I had an eighty-something former client now living in Florida email to say, "Thank you," and that she still eats and lives the way I taught her. When she came to me, she was a proverbial 'basket case' who couldn't think her way out of the proverbial paper bag. Six weeks after being on my *natural* nutrition program, she was filing her husband's and her long form federal income taxes.

The most humbling experience I had was when a client who was scheduled for a liver transplant in the early 1980s showed up at my front door carrying the largest bouquet of flowers I'd ever seen along with her daughter who used to bring her to me and her not-yet-born granddaughter to say thank you and that she didn't have the liver transplant and still has her original liver she was born with. Need I tell you how emotional a visit that was for all of us?

I share these stories because the body truly is the most magnificent piece of machinery ever invented. Its innate intelligence is far superior to what the latest science thinks it knows about the body and whose secrets it tries to reconfigure, especially with regard to human DNA. The body knows; we just have to work with it; get the toxic pollutants out, and it can do the rest, I truly believe. My professional career has proved that to me thousands of times. So, is there any reason why I would not have chosen to take the route I have for my right breast problem?

When I shared my problem with some of my colleagues, I cannot tell you the unbelievably uplifting, helpful, caring emails I received from so many. I affectionately referred to them as 'love letters'. One, in particular, that I would like to share is from Dr Rima E Laibow, MD, who has practiced holistic medicine her entire career. Dr Laibow is in Panama, Central America, and also is very active as a holistic healthcare advocate and champion.

Dr Rima E Laibow's Email

Congratulations, Catherine, not only on the emerging clinical outcome (gratifying - but predictable - as it is) but for two acts of courage for which I commend you as a physician who has spent 41 years treating people without the use of drugs of any kind.

The first act of courage has been to steadfastly cling to what you know and believe to be true - that chemotherapy, radiation, biopsies, mammograms and the rest of the allopathic panoply of high tech, low science insanity is deadly and must be avoided if you want to get well from any chronic, degenerative disease. The rational mind shuts down when we are afraid, overwhelmed, panicked. And who, facing a diagnosis of cancer, is not afraid? So when you chose the effective, but counter culture, of natural treatment for the immune system failure you are now curing (yes, curing!), you are pushing panic and irrationality aside, despite the spotless white coats of the deluded or greedy "advisors" who would propel you into the system and their well-crafted, but deadly message.

The second act of courage is to share your diagnosis, your condition and your choices openly, helping to create the community of opinion and role-modeled action which is so necessary to assist people in moving away from the deadly "official" course of action proposed and demanded of them by their doctors, insurance companies, friends, families and anyone else who presumes to press a conventional treatment model on option-seeking persons. And then, going further, making that course of treatment and choice of direction transparent to us all is a gift you are giving to us through your scholarship, analysis and writing.

Bravo, Catherine, Well Done, and Thank You!

Please know that I am available for whatever assistance you need that I can provide from this remove, since I am in Panama helping to create, among other things, an advanced medical center where the treatments like the ones you are engaged in will be available under my personal medical supervision.

Given their way, of course, the Powers That Be will make the choices you are making today illegal tomorrow in the US. They have very nearly accomplished their goals so that the treatments which you are seeking are getting harder and harder to select legally in the US and EU, making centers like the one we are creating here vitally important to health and freedom to make our own decisions and chart our own heath course, exactly as you are doing.

You are a brave woman, friend and colleague and I am proud to know you.

Yours in health and freedom,
Dr Rima
Rima E Laibow, MD
Medical Director
Natural Solutions Foundation
<DrRima.net>

Thank you, Dr Rima. I truly appreciate your kind sentiments. I wish blessings upon your work in Panama.

Doctor William G Kracht, DO, is my CAM physician managing my protocol that we have designed together. That was one of the criteria for my choosing and working with him, as I wanted to have as much input as possible into my program.

I am eternally grateful to Dr Kracht for his medical knowledge, expertise, dedication, and being there for me when I needed a physician like him to guide me through the greatest challenge of my life. Thank you, my dear Dr Kracht. I hope your wife doesn't mind my saying, "I love you."

Dr William G Kracht, DO
Catherine's Physician

Catherine Frompovich offers us an inspiring book on her story with breast cancer. Her narrative is both science-based and compelling to anyone interested in exploring natural ways to address breast cancer.

Those who are asking for breast cancer treatment options will find A Cancer Answer a very valuable resource. Catherine clearly sets a leading example to help others evaluate their cancer treatment decisions. As she states in this book, cancer is a word, not a sentence.

Why would I include material by a veterinarian in a book on female breast cancer, you probably will be asking? Well, it has to do with breast cancer in animals, and our pets in particular, because there are some definite parallels, I think. See what you think.

One of the areas of healthcare research I've been involved in since the 1980s is vaccine related adverse reactions and damage to infants, children, and adults. However, little did I realize that other health professionals like veterinarians are equally aware of and concerned about the rising problems with vaccines given to our beloved pets. Dr Patricia Jordan is one such veterinarian with whom I am in thorough agreement. Dr Patricia sends me almost daily vaccine information, studies, and other data regarding both humans and animals. When I told her about my problem and this book, she shared with me an article she had written regarding breast cancer in pets, which she thought could interest me. It did! I asked her permission to include it in my book, as I think it speaks volumes about connecting dots for cancer patients both human and pets. Thank you, Dr Jordan, for your wonderful caring.

Dr Patricia Jordan, DVM, CVA, CTCVH & Herbology
Cancer in our Pet Population
Why is it on the rise?
Dogs...Naturally! January/February 2010
Permission obtained from Dr Jordan

According to Dr Jordan,

...[A] review of the pet insurance records did show that of the four most common cancer in humans-breast, lung, prostate and colon, **only breast cancer was common in dogs.** *Breast cancer occurs in cats less frequently than in dogs but when it does is > 90% malignant adenocarcinoma.* [CJF emphasis added]

For animals the most common tumors are soft tissue sarcomas, for example, in muscles, joint tissues and nerves. While the most common cancer in our companion animals, soft tissue sarcomas are found in less than 1 % of the human cancer patients. So, what are the differences between people and their pets? ...

In many discussions, the cause of any cancer is unknown, as in human breast cancer. In 95% of human breast cancer cases the etiology or cause of the cancer remains unknown. However, the cause of soft tissue sarcomas in animals is now, well studied and now understood. The resultant findings of the Feline Vaccine Sarcoma Task Force show a clear correlation to vaccine administration and cancer formation. [CJF emphasis added]

In 1999 the WHO named the veterinary vaccine adjuvant **a grade 3 out of 4 carcinogen, with 4 being the most carcinogenic.** *The adjuvant identified is* **aluminum hydroxide**, *a* *component of most of the currently used veterinary vaccines.* **An adjuvant used also in human vaccines.** [This is most important information since many vaccines for infants, toddlers, and adults contain aluminum hydroxide, e.g., Anthrax, DTaP, DTaP-HepB-IPV, Td (Massachusetts), Hepatitis A, Hepatitis A-Hepatitis B, Hepatitis B, Tdap.] [CJF emphasis added]

Adjuvant is not the only way to transmutate a body's genome. Environmental poisons and toxins, viral oncogenes, proteins, drugs, nutritional deficiencies, hormones or mimickers and disruptors of hormones, geophysical forces, ultraviolet radiation, electro-magnetic forces, we are finding out thousands of ways to cause genetic mutation. Protecting one's DNA from transmutation is a current topic of health interest. Reversing damage done to the DNA an ongoing source of research funding.

[Why do research to reverse the damage to DNA, just stop injecting and prescribing toxic substances as health enhancers, e.g., vaccines and prescription drugs along with eliminating other factors—most of which are discussed in this book? Does that make sense? But then that would throw a huge monkey wrench into the pharmaceutical industry's plans for new products, wouldn't it?]

Vaccination as we all are now aware is lacking in any scientific evidence for long term safety or studies that it does not produce chronic disease as a trade off for the missing acute disease. ***For that matter, we have no proof that the vaccines do not cause the bulk of every haywire out of control cancer cell growth that goes by unsuppressed. In this case we find the proof that vaccines can and do cause malignant cancer.*** [CJF emphasis added] …

———

Vaccination has proved to be a big business for the veterinary medical doctor and insures job security for the needle jockeys. Big Pharma and the vaccine makers also benefit, cancer treatment is big business. Having a diagnosis of cancer means expensive drugs, possibly surgery and chemotherapy if treated via conventional medicine. *Don't forget the surgeons, there has been over a 150% increase in young women diagnosed with breast cancer choosing bilateral mastectomies, the more surgically aggressive therapy.* [CJF emphasis added] …

An important paper published in the Journal of Clinical Oncology performs a met analysis entitled "The Contribution of Cytotoxic Chemotherapy in 5 year Survival in Adult Malignancies". The objective of the paper was to accurately quantify and assess the actual benefit conferred by chemotherapy in the treatment of adults with the most common malignant cancers. All three of the authors are oncologists. One of the authors is also on an official body that advises the government in Australia on the suitability and efficacy of drugs that can be listed in the national Pharmaceutical Benefits Schedule (roughly the equivalent of the United States FDA, Food and Drug Administration). ***The meticulous study determined that in Australia chemotherapy protocols were 2.3% effective and in the United States they were found to be 2.1% effective.*** [CJF emphasis added] …

One veterinary medical doctor in Norway, using a one acupoint acupuncture technique to treat malignant breast cancer with over 75% success, has found that recovered cancer patients have approximately 12 substances in their blood, peptides that was not found in the blood of non recovered patients. His passion to follow this treatment option out met with little interest from the pharmaceutical companies. He had to self finance the testing of the substances. The substances are more effective in stopping growth in even in the Tamoxifen resistant breast cell cultures. How much money could be made off the use of the acupuncturist administering a one needle technique? The substances in the blood of the woman receiving the acupuncture treatment are of great scientific importance; after all we are talking about the successful treatment of malignant cancer!

If vaccines were not dangerous with adverse reactions and devastating health consequences, then they would not have originated a National Vaccine Injury Compensation Act. ... What needs to happen is that not only vaccine injury needs to be recognized and acknowledged, it needs to be re-ported. ...

The treatment of cancer is not likely to be found in conventional medicine. The multilevel multifactorial causation made complex by the medical industrial complex will not find the answer. Conventional wisdom will not allow conventional medicine to find an answer to cancer because it would not be profitable to do so. As said by Albert Einstein "We can't solve problems with the same thinking that created the problems". ...

A wholistic approach is needed in order to address the disease in the "whole" population. TCM [Traditional Chinese Medicine] ***and Homeopathy are two important medical systems that attest to the presentation of the "individual". Using an Integrative approach is also necessary. Only integrative practitioners integrate the being back into the mind-body-spirit trilogy of its personal picture and therefore it's***

individual expression of this biological conflict. [CJF emphasis added] …

The veterinary profession can and needs to make the right directional move on this vaccine debacle. To ignore this issue is to commit malpractice. …

[It seems like veterinary medicine finds itself in the same pickle as allopathic medicine with regard to humans, i.e., the tail wagging the dog—pardon the pun—but the pharmaceutical industry is the propelling force in both human and animal healthcare paradigms and there are similar health problems that parallel both humans and their pets, which Dr Jordan rightfully equates with the vaccine debacle the World Health Organization (WHO) apparently pointed out in 1999 regarding the veterinary vaccine adjuvant aluminum hydroxide, but no one wants to pay attention, especially Big Pharma.]

**Always keep your face turned toward
the sunny side of life.**

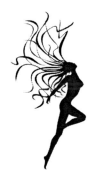

Chapter Forty-Seven
Breast Cancer Survivors

If you're going through hell, keep going.

… Sir Winston Churchill (1874—1965)
British statesman

reast cancer does not discriminate insofar as who contracts that disease.

This list, nonetheless, proves YOU can beat it!

Thanks to *Wikipedia* for this list, which you can visit at <en.wikipedia.org/wiki/List_of_breast_cancer_patients_by_survival_status>

Alive Survivors of *Female* Breast Cancer
Barbara Allen, American politician, Kansas state senator
Anastacia, American popular singer
Anita Doth, Popular Eurodance singer from the band 2 Unlimited
Christina Applegate, American television actress
Dame Eileen Atkins, British stage and film actress

Kaye Ballard, American actress and singer

Brigitte Bardot, French actress and animal rights activist

Alexandra Bastedo, British model and actress

Pat Battle, African-American news reporter and anchor for NBC News

Allyce Beasley, American actress

Jami Bernard, American author and film critic for the *New York Daily News*

Shirley Temple Black, American Oscar-winning child actress and former United States Ambassador to Ghana and Czechoslovakia, who is said to have been the first famous person to publicly announce her breast cancer diagnosis

Raelene Boyle, Australian athlete

Rhona Brankin, British politician, Member of the Scottish Parliament

Nancy Brinker, American founder of the *Susan G. Komen for the Cure*

Edna Campbell, African-American professional basketball star

Robin Carnahan, American politician, former Missouri Secretary of State

Diahann Carroll, African-American actress, singer

Agnes Chan, Asian singer and performer

Beth Nielsen Chapman, American singer-songwriter

Lois Chiles, American actress

Mary Jo Codey, former First Lady of New Jersey

Sheryl Crow, American singer/musician

Pat Danner, American politician; former Democratic U.S. House Representative from Missouri

Ruby Dee, African-American stage and film actress
Diana Dill, British-American actress; ex-wife of American actor
Kirk Douglas; mother of American actor Michael Douglas
Anita Doth, Eurodance singer from the Dutch duo 2 Unlimited
Susan Duncan, Australian author
Barbara Ehrenreich, American author/ethicist
Jill Eikenberry, American actress
Linda Ellerbee, American television correspondent/journalist
Melissa Etheridge, American singer; lesbian activist
Marianne Faithfull, British singer and actress
Edie Falco, American film, stage and television actress
Rita Fan Hsu Lai-tai, Hong Kong politician and Honorary
President of the Hong Kong Breast Cancer Foundation
Catherine Drew Gilpin Faust, American academic, historian,
and current (as of 2009) President of Harvard University
Deanna Favre, founded The Deanna Favre Hope Foundation
and wife of American football quarterback Brett Favre
Carly Fiorina, American entrepreneur and 2010 California
Republican political candidate for the United States Senate
Caitlin Flanagan, American magazine writer, editor and book
author
Peggy Fleming, American figure skater
Maria Friedman, British actress
Liza Goddard, British actress
Nanci Griffith, American singer/songwriter
Dorothy Hamill, American Olympic champion figure skater
Jane Hamsher, American film producer, author and liberal
blogger

Sheila Hancock, British stage and film actress

Julie Harris, American film, stage and television actress

Heidi Heitkamp, North Dakota politician and lawyer

Marsha Hunt, African-American singer, novelist, breast cancer activist and mother of Mick Jagger's first child, Karis Jagger

Laura Ingraham, American radio host/pundit

Kate Jackson, American film and television actress

Ann Jillian, American film, television and musical theatre actress

Betsey Johnson, American fashion designer

Melanie Johnson, former British Member of Parliament

Susan Kadis, Canadian politician in the Canadian House of Commons

Vera Katz, American politician (first woman Speaker of the Oregon House of Representatives; 45th mayor of Portland, Oregon)

Maeve Kinkead, American soap opera and television actress

Hoda Kotb, Egyptian-American television news anchor, journalist and correspondent

Peggy Lautenschlager, American politician from the state of Wisconsin

Marilyn Lloyd, member of the U.S. House of Representatives who was diagnosed with breast cancer, was denied a silicone breast implant following her treatment because the U.S. Food and Drug Administration had removed them from the market, and became an advocate for legislation related to breast cancer treatment and women's health

Geralyn Lucas, American journalist, television producer, and writer

Marisa Acocella Marchetto, American writer, cartoonist and memoirist

Judy Eason McIntyre, African-American politician; Oklahoma State Senator

Amanda Mealing, British television and soap opera actress

Wendy Mesley, Canadian host and reporter for CBC Television

Kylie Minogue, Australian singer, actress

Mary Ann Mobley, American actress, musician, and activist; Miss America 1959

Hala Moddelmog, American president and CEO of *Susan G. Komen for the Cure*

Diana Moran, British model, fitness expert and journalist

Shelley Morrison, American film and television actress; also battled lung cancer

Jenni Murray, British BBC presenter

Sue Myrick, American politician, Republican U.S. House Representative from North Carolina

Janet Napolitano, American politician and current (as of 2010) United States Secretary of Homeland Security; former Governor of Arizona

Kitten Natividad, Mexican adult film actress and model

Jocelyn Newman, former Senator from the Australian Parliament for Tasmania; treated successfully

Phyllis Newman, American television and musical theatre actress, singer

Olivia Newton-John, UK/Australian singer/actress

Cynthia Nixon, American stage, film and television actress
Linda Nolan, Irish-born singer, actress and former member of the 1970s pop band, The Nolans
Kim Novak, American film actress
Sandra Day O'Connor, first woman United States Supreme Court justice
Elaine Paige, English musical theatre actress, singer
Nancy Priddy, mother of American actress Christina Applegate
Judy Rankin, American Hall of Fame professional golfer
Betsy Rawls, American Hall of Fame professional golfer
Nancy Reagan, former U.S. First Lady
M. Jodi Rell, American politician, Governor of Connecticut
Cokie Roberts, American journalist
Robin Roberts, African-American women's basketball player, ESPN sportscaster
Margaretta Fitler Murphy Rockefeller aka Happy Rockefeller, American socialite and wife of former N.Y. Governor and U.S. Vice President Nelson Rockefeller
Betty Rollin, American author, retired TV
Debbie Wasserman Schultz, American politician; United States House Representative from the 20th District of Florida and chairwoman of the Democratic National Committee
Debra Shipley, British politician; Labour Party member of Parliament
Claire Shulman, former Borough President of Queens, New York City
Carly Simon, American singer
Jaclyn Smith, American actress, businesswoman

Dame Maggie Smith, Oscar-winning British actress of stage and screen

Suzanne Somers, American television actress and personality

Karin Stanford, African-American professor and writer

Koo Stark, American former adult film actress

Gloria Steinem, American feminist activist

Lynne Stewart, American lawyer/activist

Ruth Ann Swenson, American soprano opera star

Stephanie Swift, American adult film actress

Maura Tierney, American film and television actress

Jools Topp, New Zealand folk singer, one of the Topp Twins

Linda Tripp, former United States government federal employee who played a significant role in the impeachment proceedings against then President Bill Clinton

Dawn Upshaw, American opera singer

Ann Veneman, former head of the U.S. Dept. of Agriculture

Joyce Wadler, American journalist, writer and memoirist (surviving ovarian cancer as well)

Liza Wang, Hong Kong television actress and personality, singer and diva

Linda Waterfall, American singer-songwriter

Courtesy *Wikipedia's* Creative Commons Attribution-ShareAlike License

The above women have celebrity. However, there are thousands—maybe hundreds of thousands—of women breast

cancer survivors whose names are not listed here. I honor them too.

❧

These are some of the bravest women you may ever meet. I salute them.

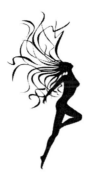

Epilogue
The Author's **Opinionated** *Observations*

*Never lose trust in your body that the power of an illness, e.g.,
breast cancer, appears to be greater than your body's ability for
healing. Remember with Creator God all things are possible when
you know and honor His ways. Nature is One of His Ways.*

... Catherine J Frompovich

Somehow after years of working in consumer health research and writing about it, plus what I've been learning with my right breast odyssey, I'm left with the feeling that the allopathic cancer establishment puts full faith and trust in toxic modalities that for some patients cause more harm as opposed to supporting the body's inborn, Creator-given capacity to heal with natural substances the body knows how to use for millennial generations. Theirs, I believe, is an exclusive prejudice against anything except 'cut, burn, and poison' treatments they call the 'gold standard'.

Since I've been on this odyssey I've seen, heard, and learned a lot—maybe more than I wanted to know. Every story I've heard stupefies me more than the previous one. When you sit for about two hours taking an intravenous drip of vitamin C every week, you come to hear overwhelmingly sad stories of how people were 'taken for a ride', I'd say, by the allopathic cancer establishment only to be told, "There's nothing more we can do; go home and get your affairs in order." So many cancer patients have landed in that sad state, and only then, when given a short period of time to live diagnosis, do they decide to turn to holistic cancer treatment. What amazes me is that if they found complementary cancer treatment so late, how come they did not find it sooner before their body had been mutilated, burned, and poisoned by surgery, radiation, and chemotherapy.

One time I heard the pathetic story of a gentleman who had rectal cancer surgery and while surgeons were in there, they found it spread so they took care of his prostate; subjected him to radiation and, of course, chemotherapy. He said what he went through from the surgery alone took him over two months to feel no surgical pains, but then he had to deal with radiation sickness and the after effects of harsh chemotherapy. Then, what really bothered him most of all, was when he was told, "There's nothing more we can do for you; go home and get your affairs in order." What devastation!

Stories like that prompt my mind to question why any patient would allow the allopathic cancer establishment to get into your head and scare you into such harsh treatments. I only can imagine what that gentleman heard from his surgeon and oncologist upon his initial visit(s). All the scare talk they give and then, when patients buy into it, they most often contract secondary cancers down the timeline, or are abandoned with no hope from 'gold standard' treatments that health insurance companies pay mega bucks to support and perpetuate, it seems.

Shortly before finishing writing this book I heard the extremely sad story about an individual who contracted leukemia and went the conventional allopathic cancer treatment route of having the immune system destroyed with chemotherapy drugs so that a bone marrow transplant could be done. Need I tell you how the family frantically searched for a bone marrow match. After one had been located, the appointed time came for the immune system 'kill' followed by the transplant.

I cannot tell you how the patient's family hoped and prayed for success. Unfortunately, within less than a month the patient was dead. How devastating to everyone. But that got me to thinking, so please pardon what I say next, as it may sound a little brash.

Allopathic medicine *deliberately destroys* the immune system, the patient dies, and that seems to be okay within the medical profession and society in general—if not accepted as a norm when things go wrong and health insurance pays for it. There are no accusations of quackery, no claims the protocol doesn't work, or that their methods kill—none of that is to be heard anywhere, whereas in reality, it's patently true, I think.

Being a person who likes to deal from the top of the deck, what do you think would have happened had that same patient died while undergoing holistic cancer treatments?

That patient's death probably would have been included in some "quack hunter's" database as another victim killed by holistic, complementary and alternative medicine (CAM). Do you think I'm mistaken or exaggerating? I don't think so. There truly is a double standard.

My take on that leukemia patient—now deceased—is that 'they' probably would still be alive with an immune system still intact and working because it would have been supported, enhanced, and uplifted—*not deliberately destroyed.* Since the immune system is the body's prime defense mechanism in battling any disease, especially cancer, why destroy it? Good question? But, in my opinion, allopathic medicine can get away with *its brand of legal quackery* that is accepted as the 'gold standard' and for which insurance companies, in essence, 'pay to kill'. That really doesn't make sense, does it?

Here's the kicker: Even though I'm paying for my treatments out of pocket, I have spent about 15 percent of what standard chemotherapy treatments *alone* would cost. I have not included the costs insurance companies would have paid for radiation, surgery, and diagnostic procedures. If I included them, I guess my costs so far would be about 1 to 2 percent of the standard allopathic breast cancer protocols. Also, I am functioning very well, have not been sick, and the tumors are greatly reduced. See the end of my comments in this *Epilogue* for a surprise.

Cancer apparently results from the ultimate of toxic insults to the body's immune system, which had been attacked and overcome by any number or combinations of physiological and/or emotional insults including—but not limited to—those in the environment, food growing and processing industries, chemicals, fluoride, pesticides, pharmaceuticals including vaccines, nuclear power plants regularly releasing radioactive particulates into the air, toxic chemicals and metals that make up chemtrails crisscrossing the sky to control weather patterns since 1999, and all the electromagnetic frequencies from cell phones to TVs to computers to microwave ovens to WiFi to—you name it, and last but not least, genetics.

However, nothing may add more onslaughts and insults to the human immune system's breakdown than the medical industry with all their high tech electronic nuclear scans, plus tracer and imaging 'cocktails' that one is given either to drink or have injected into one's body. For each CT, MRI, mammogram, and X-ray the human body retains cumulative radiation and/or chemical damage, and yet doctors write scripts for these tests without batting an eyelash, it seems. How did they practice medicine before such technologies? And seemingly there were less dramatically ill people in the 1950s, 1960s, and 1970s.

Part of the problem, I think, is the acculturation process by which advertisements program consumers that being sick or unhealthy is normal and to be expected. Just listen to radio ads; watch TV; or read a magazine, and one is overwhelmed with propaganda and hype about the state of the art of medicine practiced in doctors' offices and special hospitals. Just about everywhere one looks, there's a reminder of sickness or a threat about contracting some disease. In essence, everyone is pre-programmed.

In my opinion, the allopathic medical community plays a contributory role in the world of cancer since they prescribe and make mega bucks from modalities that have built-in side effects that are played down and can result in secondary cancers. For example, how many scans, X-rays, and imagings do you think are prescribed *a year* in the USA?

According to the U.S. CDC's ***National Ambulatory Medical Care Survey: 2008 Summary Tables, Table 17*** there were

Tests or Imagings	Listed in thousands
Mammograms	21,069
X-rays	58,184
CTs (computed tomography scans)	15,247
MRIs (magnetic resonance imaging	15,479
Totals for any imaging	146,453

As confirmed by the U.S. CDC on its website <cdc.gov/nchs/data/ahcd/names_summary/namessum2008.pdf>

Incidentally, I'm not the only one who questions such exposures. Back on September 29, 2009 *CBS News* website posted an article by Jonathan LaPook titled, "Too Many Unnecessary MRIs and CT Scans?" that cited these statistics:

> ***CT scans are big money makers, costing anywhere from $300 to $1,000. MRIs run as high as $1300.*** [126]

The annual price tag for imaging? $100 billon. And experts estimate 35 percent of these tests aren't even necessary. That's potentially $35 billion wasted every year. [126] [CJF emphasis added]

Did you by chance catch the amount of money "wasted?" What does that tell you? How does that impact the spiraling costs of healthcare plus residual and secondary *iatrogenic* health problems?

In September 2011 *Kaiser Health News* website 'shouted' "Concern Is Growing That The Elderly Get Too Many Medical Tests" in which

> *Dartmouth physician Lisa M. Schwartz cites one such case: a healthy 78-year-old man who was left incontinent and impotent by radiation treatments for prostate cancer, a disease that typically grows so slowly that many men die with – but not of – it.* [127]

How about this?

> *While cancer screenings are most common, other tests are overused among the elderly, Klein and others say. They include cholesterol testing, which can lead to the prescription of statin drugs that require regular blood tests to check liver function; typically, cholesterol plaque takes years to accumulate, and statins confer only a modest benefit in the elderly. Likewise, CT scans of the heart or whole body can*

unearth suspicious findings, such as lung nodules, which trigger a painful and risky lung biopsy, but often turn out to be benign. [127]

One quotation from that *Kaiser Health News* website really stands out for me, and it comes from Lisa M Schwartz, MD, professor at the Dartmouth Institute for Health Policy and Clinical Practice:

"...But we never seem to talk about the downside of testing."

Some allopathic physicians, who themselves have experienced cancer, change their opinion about standard allopathic cancer treatment and go the holistic route. Dr Servan-Schreiber's story [now deceased] is a fascinating read about his twenty-year battle with brain cancer. Please visit online <anti-cancerbook.com/>.

On Dr Schreiber's website, these profound statements appear:

Why the traditional Western diet creates the conditions for disease and how to develop a science-based anticancer diet [to which I'd like to say, the diet in the book you are reading does just that—*creates an anti-cancer diet*—by favorably adjusting pH and saturating nutrient content to effectively negate and reprogram cancer-producing conditions]

How and why sugar and stress feed cancer and ways to achieve life balance and good nutrition to combat it [This book's chapters on diet and nutrition explain what Dr Schreiber is alluding to.]

How to minimize environmental toxins [If you want a detailed discourse on how to do that, may I suggest reading my last book, *Our Chemical Lives And the Highjacking of Our DNA* available on Amazon.com.]

How to find the right blend of traditional and alternative health care [as far as this author is concerned, that just may not be possible until allopathic medicine realizes that it does not have *all the answers* to dealing with breast cancer—or any type of cancer for that matter—and becomes more humble and willing in its approach to accepting that it must stop acting like a schoolyard bully regarding holistic, alternative, complementary healthcare and cancer treatment modalities. That would include the AMA and FDA, too, in my opinion.]

To put things into proper perspective, please consider that a top executive of GlaxoSmithKline, who happened to be their worldwide vice president of genetics, candidly admitted, *"The vast majority of drugs—more than 90 percent—only work in 30 to 50 percent of the people."* Chemotherapy is a drug—a high-priced one at that. So what that really means is that much of what is promoted and sold as 'miracle medicine'—prescription drugs and chemotherapy—does not work for most people— and in essence may be wasted healthcare insurance expenditures. What a waste of money and resources, I'd say. By the way, it was Dr Allen Roses, MD, then senior vice-president of genetics research at GlaxoSmithKline, who made that rather revealing statement.

After reading this book you probably think there's so much you don't know, and are asking why? Perhaps the paper "Modern Medicine is not a science" by Dr Vernon Coleman online at <whale.to/a/coleman3.html> can help you understand the *raison d'être*. Dr Coleman's other paper, "The Real Cause of Cancer And the Solution," which is online at <whale.to/cancer/coleman.html>, may shed more light on the politics of cancer and why a cure never may be found. Candidly, Dr Coleman writes, *"The most repressive, most prejudiced and most obscenely intolerant branch of the international medical industry is undoubtedly that part of it which claims to deal with cancer."*

So, is there a particular panacea? Maybe not! However, there should be enforced rights and respect for patients to chose what they want as their healthcare and not be hounded or disenfranchised from healthcare insurance reimbursement because of their choices and their inherent rights to self-determination for themselves and their children. Based upon my experience and example, health insurers could be saving a helluva lot of money if they were more in line with having breast cancer patients treated holistically—but that's my opinion.

Please keep in mind that when breast cancer is stabilized—the tumor has been reduced even less than 50 percent in size and not metastasizing—some women can live twenty or more years with tumors that are stabilized. That's important information to know and strive to achieve. Please read that again. However, to attain that status, you must be committed to sticking with a treatment regimen that keeps it stabilized, and holistic breast management offers that, I feel, as opposed to being made toxic and terribly sick with increased chances of secondary cancers or hearing from your oncologist, "There's nothing more we can do for you; get your affairs in order."

One thing we all must remember, though, is *even when we are cured of cancer*, we still will die some day from something, perhaps a car accident or some other freak event. No one gets off the planet alive, but the way in which we make the transition can be influenced by our wants, needs, desires, personal preference, and choices about medical-induced suffering, I truly believe. Personally, I don't want treatments that border on the chamber of horrors stories. And neither do a lot of women. From what I've gathered, close to 80 percent of USA-treated cancer patients say they have used some form of holistic, complementary and alternative medicine (CAM) treatment. What is that telling you?

There's a significant and possibly *elegant* philosophy that I'd like to share regarding life in general and one's health, in particular. I truly believe if it's our time to go, nothing—including allopathic medicine's greatest advances—will buy us a moment of time—since that's what transitioning is all about: Going home—back to where we came from.

May I share with you how I blew the breast surgeon's mind with my answer when I was being 'read the riot act' about getting the 'gold standard' treatment and not to go the holistic route? I said as gently, but as firmly, as I could enunciate, *"Doctor, the way I see it, it's a win-win situation. If I beat it— and I know I will—I've won. If I don't and transition back home, then I've also won because I will be in a better place than where*

I am now. So, I'm not afraid." At that point I think the doctor knew that my head was on straight about not living with medical fear or guilt.

I certainly don't regret the route I have taken. My last evaluation was April 27, 2012 shortly before I finished editing this book. This is what I emailed my friends and colleagues about that evaluation:

> *Today I had a 4-month evaluation and progress report on my R breast problem that I am managing totally holistically. After an examination my managing holistic physician declared that there was a lot gone, but what remained, was very soft and broken up to which I say, "Thank God" and thanks to all who have sent me their prayers and good wishes, which I totally appreciate and value.*
>
> *FYI: There were two tumors that protruded out of the breast the size of half a large orange. The R breast now looks like the Left. However, I've had no mammograms, just thermogram and 2 sonograms; no chemotherapy nor chemo pills, no radiation, no biopsies, no mastectomy, no radiation sickness, no nerve damage, no "chemo brain."*

Now I will reveal the readings from the *"US Breast Bilateral – Aug 1 2011 2:22 PM Ultrasound examination of both breast"* performed in the Department of Radiology at a hospital and medical center.

> *Examination of the right breast reveals a prominent irregular shadowing mass in the 10:00 position approximately*

4 to 5 cm from the nipple. This measures up to 2.0x 2.8 x 3.1 cm.

In the 11:00 position approximately 4-5 cm is also an echogenic area which may be somewhat spiculated measuring 2.3 x 1.7 x 2.0 cm. This may extend in Cooper's ligaments. Both areas are suspicious for neoplasm. ...

Indication: Palpable mass, abnormal thermogram

Highly suggestive of malignancy. Appropriate action should be taken.

Notation by the sonogram-evaluating MD: *We do have a copy of a thermogram study of both breasts dated July 26, 2011.*

I personally spoke with the patient and she is aware of the current findings. She does not wish to have any additional imaging studies such as mammography.

Oh, by the way, this is what the ultrasound found regarding my left breast:

Survey scanning the left breast revealed no discrete findings.

So you see it was not my imagination, not an "all in my head nightmare;" it was and is real. I plan on having another sonogram and thermogram when my managing physician and I feel there is nothing more to palpate. I've come a long way in just ten exciting and life-altering months. My last blood tests taken four days after my last evaluation were *EXCELLENT!*

I'm stress-free and that's a wonderful feeling, plus empowering. As I tell everyone, *"Don't let them get into your head and own you. It's your body; it's your choice."*

Ralph Waldo Emerson, years ago said something so elegant, I think, that I want to use his beautiful prose to end this book:

> *To laugh often and much; to win the respect of intelligent people and the affection of children; to earn the appreciation of honest critics and endure the betrayal of false friends; to appreciate beauty; to find the best in others; to leave the world a bit better whether by a healthy child, a garden patch, or a redeemed social condition; to know even one life has breathed easier because you have lived. This is to have succeeded.*

By writing *A Cancer Answer* I hope I have brought some sanity and a sense of helpful humaneness along with some Light to the treatment and management of a disease that's afflicting over 230,000 *female* and over 2,000 *male breast cancer patients* in the USA just in 2011, according to the National Cancer Institute. Now multiply that by each succeeding year. This is a war we just have to win. *We can when we womanize the battlements to our wants and needs.* I hope and pray this book will help set the course to humane breast cancer treatment for women everywhere.

The Ultimate in After Thoughts

Shortly before completing the book you are reading, I came across some information that just about blew my mind insofar as it emphasized, confirmed, and reiterated all that I believe about healing cancer, have known, am doing, and have written about in this book.

What I'm referring to is an article in the December 2011 issue of the *Noetic Now Journal* by researcher Kelly A Turner, PhD, titled "When Cancer Disappears: The Curious Phenomenon of 'Unexpected Remission'" published by the Institute of Noetic Sciences at <noetic.org/noetic/issue-seventeen-december/unexpected-remission>. Dr Kelly is a researcher, lecturer, and consultant in the field of Integrative Oncology.

Basically what Dr Kelly confirms is of absolute importance in a holistic approach to managing, treating, and healing cancer of any type—and breast cancer, in particular, I would add.

Dr Kelly's research took her around the globe interviewing numerous healers and patients, and she came up with the following, which I have known about since the 1980s and convinced me of my beliefs about dealing with cancer:

- Changing one's diet
- Experiencing a deepening spirituality
- Feeling Love/Joy/Happiness
- Releasing repressed emotions
- Taking herbs or vitamins
- Taking control of health decisions
- Having a strong will to live
- Receiving social support

all of which I discuss in exciting and workable detail together with much, much more that I believe works to make the healing process effective, timely, and permanent.

I express my most sincere thanks to Dr Kelly for her innovative research and publishing it in an extremely insightful article, which I truly hope allopathic medicine will take seriously and implement. I also have another suggestion for the cancer establishment and that is to take *this* book seriously, as it offers what your breast cancer patients need to get well.

Catherine's Most Recent Update

As the galleys for this book were being proofed, I had a right breast sonogram performed at a hospital. The results confirm that the holistic program and protocols I am using, as discussed in this book, work. The sonogram measurements for the tumors now read .06 cm and 1.1 cm. *Hallelujah!*

Catherine J Frompovich

Appendix A

The 'Unknown' About Polio Vaccine: SV40 and Cancer

By Catherine J. Frompovich | April 9th, 2011 | Category: By Author, Catherine Frompovich, Top Stories | 10 comments

*A*fter half a century, the 108th U.S. Congress House of Representatives Subcommittee on Human Rights and Wellness finally held a hearing September 10, 2003, on the simian virus (SV40) that was included in the original polio vaccine produced and administered to children in the 1950s and 1960s.

Candidly, the first page of the transcript for the hearing states:

There is no dispute that millions of Americans received polio vaccines that were contaminated with the virus called Simian Virus 40, or SV–40. There also is no dispute that SV–40 is capable of causing cancer, but there is a major dispute as to how many Americans may have received the contaminated vaccine, with estimates ranging from 4 million to 100 million people. There is also a major dispute as to when the polio vaccine supply got cleaned up. In addition, nobody knows how many people got sick or died because of the contaminated vaccines.

In his opening statement, Subcommittee Chairman Dan Burton reiterated:

But there is a major dispute as to how many Americans may have received the contaminated vaccine with estimates ranging from 4 million to 100 million. There is also a major dispute as to when the polio vaccine supply got cleaned-up. In addition, nobody knows how many people got sick or died because of the contaminated vaccines.

One of the experts who testified, James Goedert, MD, said:

The virus was discovered in 1960 in rhesus macaque monkey kidney cells that were used in the production of the original Salk and Sabin polio vaccines (1). Since the mass immunization program for polio began in 1955, before the discovery of the virus, contaminated vaccine lots were inadvertently used for the first few years of the program.

Dr. Goedert went on to say that, "**...no SV40 has been found in U.S. polio vaccine lots tested after 1972.**"

He further added that **"The Institute of Medicine (IOM) of the National Academy of Sciences issued a report in October 2002 (50), which concluded that scientific 'evidence is inadequate to accept or reject a causal relationship between SV40-containing polio vaccines and cancer.' (p.11, Executive Summary). The committee stated that the 'biological evidence is of moderate strength that SV40 exposure could lead to cancer in humans under natural conditions' and that 'biological evidence is of moderate strength that SV40 exposure from the polio vaccine is related to SV40 infection in humans.'"** (p. 11, Executive Summary)

Barbara Loe Fisher, of the National Vaccine Information Center, testified at that hearing and here's part of what she had to say:

The story you're about to hear involves a pharmaceutical company which used monkeys to make polio vaccine, government health agencies responsible for making sure the vaccine was not contaminated with monkey viruses, and individuals who are now dying from cancerous tumors that contain a monkey virus which appears to have contaminated that polio vaccine. At the heart of this story is a violation of the public trust and the informed consent ethic.

Ms. Fisher's last sentence still holds true today: At the heart of the vaccine/vaccination safety issue is "**a violation of the public trust and informed consent ethic.**" Informed consent is becoming more problematic—if not totally lacking—because dozens more vaccines are being mandated by health agencies and an irresponsibly administered U.S. CDC and FDA that parrot vaccine makers' pseudo-science about neurotoxins and other poisons in vaccines. The SV40 issue should make everyone question IF vaccine makers really know what they are doing. And still, parents are mandated by state laws to have their children harmed and/or killed from unproven or even unknown ingredients—as SV40 proved—in vaccines.

Furthermore, Ms. Fisher pointed out that

There is frank admission that the limitations of technology and lack of scientific knowledge means there can be no guarantee that vaccines will not be contaminated with substances that could prove harmful to humans 1 day.

Nothing is more indicative of Ms. Fisher's statement than all the foreign DNA that is used in the manufacture of vaccines now in the 21st century. According to CDC's **Adjuvant,**

Excipient, and Medium Summary, there is bovine and bovine calf, chick, human diploid tissue (aborted human fetuses), African green monkey, mouse brain, and Rhesus monkey just to mention a few. Just recently insects were added to the mix.

During testimony, Stanley P. Kops, Esquire, presented stunning charts of facts about SV40 and challenged the polio vaccine maker to dispute them with pharma's corroborating facts or evidence. Kops's presentation also noted that the vaccine maker did not follow the mandatory **Code of Federal Regulations**, plus he supplied language from a corporate interoffice memo stating that, that specific vaccine maker did not do the proper tests for extraneous agents or neurovirulence. Mr. Kops apparently acquired much of the facts/data during the discovery process in lawsuits where he represented damaged clients in court.

In 2000 Attorney Kops's article, "Oral Polio Vaccine and Human Cancer: A Reassessment of SV40 as a Contaminant Based upon Legal Documents" was published in **Anticancer Research**, pages 4745-49.

Also testifying, Adi F. Gazdar, MD, said **"…more than 60 laboratories world wide have documented the presence of SV40 in human tumors…" "The biological evidence is strong that SV40 is a cancer causing virus."**

The committee, after hearing testimony, recommended that the appropriate federal agencies develop a Vaccine Contamination Prevention and Response Plan.

The revelation that SV40—a cancer-causing virus—was in polio vaccines for numerous years without apparent detection or concern by the vaccine maker, leads one to believe that vaccine manufacturing may be nothing short of a crapshoot. Throw it together and get it out in the marketplace as soon as possible along with media spin touting that it will prevent a disease.

Sadly, the polio vaccine is not the only vaccine with problems. Just about every vaccine on the market today is problematic insofar as it contains neurotoxins and other poisons further compounded by foreign DNA that is syringed into an infant, toddler, teenager, adult, and senior citizen without much regard for adverse reactions. Too many vaccines in the past have ruined many lives with **Guillain Barré** Syndrome, a paralyzing adverse reaction to vaccines. Currently there is scientific talk about DNA from aborted fetuses being implicated in infant adverse reactions.

The CDC's VAERS reports document thousands of serious adverse reactions to vaccines, and no one seems to be connecting the dots on these ticking time bombs. Do we have to wait another fifty years to hear the facts? That leads one to think it must be deliberate because they really can't be that damn dumb.

# # #

Online available at: <vactruth.com/2011/04/09/polio-vaccine-sv40-cancer/>

Endnotes

Endnotes provide online website addresses to additional information and/or scientific documentation. LAI refers to *Last Accessed Information*, the date information was last verified during the editing process for the book.

Introduction

1. Sherrill Sellman, "Tamoxifen A Major Medical Mistake," Natural Health and Longevity Resource Center, <all-natural. com/tamox.html> LAI 4/3/12

2. Janette D Sherman, MD, "Excerpts from Chapter 9 Tamoxifen Chemical manipulation," Life's Delicate Balance. LAI 4/3/12 <alwayseco.com/Tamoxifen_janettedshermanmd.pdf>

3. MedlinePlus, "Radiation Sickness," LAI 4/3/12 <nlm.nih.gov/ medlineplus/ency/article/000026.htm>

4. Mercola.com, "The Town of Allopath," LAI 4/3/12 <mercola. com/townofallopath/index.htm>

5. Breast Cancer.Org, "U.S. Breast Cancer Statistics," LAI 4/3/12 <breastcancer.org/symptoms/understand_bc/statistics.jsp>

6. "Harold Saive presents Geoengineering Aluminum Lab Results to County Commission Public Comments on Aug. 9, 2011" LAI 4/3/12 <youtube.com/watch?feature=player_embedded &v=j42bvkFbit8>

Chapter 1

7. ScienceDaily, "Earliest Evidence Of Modern Humans Detected," Oct. 17, 2007 <sciencedaily.com/releases/2007/10/071017145252.htm> LAI 4/5/12

8. The History Channel, "12,000 Year-Old Stone Structures," LAI 4/5/12 <forbiddenknowledgetv.com/videos/ancient-civilizations/12000-year-old-stone-structures.html>

9. Wikipedia, the free encyclopedia, "Paleolithic diet," LAI 4/5/12 <en.wikipedia.org/wiki/Paleolithic_diet>

10. K Kris Hurst, "Otzi the Iceman," About.com Archaeology, LAI 4/5/12 <archaeology.about.com/od/iterms/qt/iceman.htm>

11. JR Wilt, PhD, "Biblical ills and remedies," *Journal of the Royal Society of Medicine*, Vol. 79, 1986, LAI 4/5/12 <ncbi.nlm.nih.gov/pmc/articles/PMC1290577/pdf/jrsocmed001830060.pdf>

12. Biotechnology Information Series (Bio 3) North Central Regional Extension Publication Iowa State University – University Extension. "Bovine Somatotropin (bST)" December 1993, LAI 4/5/12 <biotech.iastate.edu/biotech_info_series/Bovine_Somatotropin.html>

13. Dan Flynn, "Test Finds Too Much Juice in CA Dairy Cow," Food Safety News, Aug. 24, 2011, LAI 4/5/12 <foodsafetynews.com/2011/08/test-finds-too-much-juice-in-ca-dairy-cow>

14. Disclose.tv truth revealed, "Smart Dust Probes in Chemtrails," LAI 4/5/12 <disclose.tv/action/viewvideo/56909/Smart_Dust_Probes_In_Chemtrails/>

15. The High Frequency Active Auroral Research Program, "HAARP A Premier Facility for the Study of Ionospheric Physics and Radio Science," LAI 4/5/12

16. Hill Laboratories, Analysis Report, May 6, 2010, LAI 4/5/12 <chemtrailsnorthnz.files.wordpress.com/2010/05/788376-sp-1.pdf>

17. Elizabeth Rosenthal, "Radiation, Once Free, Can Follow Tricky Path," *The New York Times,* March 21, 2011, LAI 4/5/12 <nytimes.com/2011/03/22/science/earth/22food.html>

18. Mayo Clinic High Cholesterol, "Trans fat is double trouble for your heart health," LAI 4/5/12 <mayoclinic.com/health/trans-fat/CL00032>

19. Gary Taubes, "Is Sugar Toxic?" *The New York Times Magazine,* April 13, 2011, LAI 4/5/12 <nytimes.com/2011/04/17/magazine/mag-17Sugar-t.html?pagewanted=all>

20. Reuters, "Cancer cells slurp up fructose, US study finds," Aug. 2, 2010, LAI 4/5/12 <reuters.com/article/2010/08/02/cancer-fructose-idAFN0210830520100802>

21. "Lp2 Cancer deaths in 1970 and in 1997," LAI 4/5/12 <gilbertling.org/lp2.htm>

22. International Wellness Directory, "Cancer Loves Sugar," LAI 4/5/12 <mnwelldir.org/docs/nutrition/sugar.htm>

23. U.S. Food and Drug Administration, "Food Additive Status List," LAI 4/5/12 <fda.gov/Food/FoodIngredientsPackaging/FoodAdditives/FoodAdditiveListings/uncm091048.htm>

24. L Herber, "The Problem of Chemicals in Food," *Anarchist Archives*, LAI 4/5/12 <dwardmac.pitzer.edu/Anarchist_Archives/bookchin/HerbertChem.html>

25. Catherine J Frompovich, "Our Chemical Lives And The Hijacking Of Our DNA, A Probe Into What's Probably Making

Us Sick," <amazon.com/Our-Chemical-Lives-Hijacking-DNA/dp/1439255369> LAI 4/5/12

26. The Analyst Diagnose ME.com, "DIM (di-indolmethane) / 13C (Indole-3-Carbanol)" <diagnose-me.com/treat/T271923.html> LAI 4/7/12

27. KOPN Audio Archive, "Why and how organic agriculture CAN feed the world," Melinda Hemmelgarn / guest Jeff Moyer, LAI 4/7/12 <kopn.org/aasp?u=http://kopn.org/a/showrss4.php?n=http://kopn.org/dc/dircaster2.php?p=fs>

Chapter 2

28. Wikipedia, the free encyclopedia, "Chemical weapons in World War I," LAI 4/7/12 <en.wikipedia.org/wiki/Chemical_weapons_in_World_War_I>

29. U.S. Department of Labor, Bureau of Labor Statistics, Occupational Outlook Handbook, "Career Guide to Industries," <bls.gov/oco/cg/cgs008.htm> LAI 4/7/12

30. Mohammad H Forouzanfar, et al. "Breast and cervical cancer in 187 countries between 1980 and 2010: a systematic analysis," *The Lancet,* Vol. 378, Issue 9801, pp. 1461-1484, 22 October 2011 LAI 4/7/12 <thelancet.com/journals/lancet/article/PIIS0140-6736(11)61351-2/abstract>

31. National Breast Cancer Coalition, "Facts and Statistics about Breast Cancer in the United States:2011," LAI 4/7/12 <breastcancerdeadline2020.org/know/analyses-factsheets–other/>

32. Shelley Moore, "About Toothpaste Tubes Made of Metal," eHow health, LAI 4/7/12 <ehow.com/about_4597108_toothpaste-tubes-made-metal.html>

33. Guna Biotherapeutics, for layperson information <gunainc.com/index.php>, for healthcare professionals <gunainc.com> and sign in according to request. LAI 4/7/12

Chapter 4

34. Mayo Clinic, Breast Cancer Overview, LAI 4/7/12 <mayoclinic.org/breast-cancer/?mc_id=comlinkpilot&placement=bottom>

35. *Medscape*, "Gynecomastia," Pathologic LAI 4/7/12 <emedicine.medscape.com/article/120858-overview#aw2aab6b2b2aa>

Chapter 5

36. "Mammography: Past and Present Parts 1-8," LAI 4/7/12 <ratical.org/radiation/CNR/PBC/chp28F.html>

37. Peggy Girshman, "Mammogram Controversy: 'Politics Is Always Intruding Into The World Of Breast Cancer'," *Kaiser Health News,* Nov. 20, 2009, LAI 4/7/12 <kaiserhealthnews.org/Checking-In-With/breast-cancer-and-politics.aspx>

38. Maureen Glabman, "Lobbyists That The Founders Just Never Dreamed of," *Managed Care* Public Policy, August 2002 LAI 4/7/12 <managedcaremag.com/archives/0208/0208.lobbying.html>

39. Dan Eggen, "Lobbyists Spend Millions to Influence Health Care," *The Washington Post* Daily Dose, July 21, 2009 LAI 4/7/12 <voices.washingtonpost.com/health-care-reform/2009/07/health_care_continues_its_inte.html>

40. HealthNewsReview.Org, "WSJ follows the mammogram money & lobbying," Jan. 12, 2010, LAI 4/7/12 <healthnewsreview.org/blog/2010/01/wsj-follows-the-mammogram-money-lobbying.html>

41. Wikipedia, the free encyclopedia, "Misuse of statistics," LAI 4/7/12 <en.wikipedia.org/wiki/Misuse_of_statistics>

42. Lynn Morales, ND, *Health Choices Lead to Health Lifestyle,* "Mammogram Alternatives," LAI 4/7/12 <lynnmoralesnd.com/tag/mammogram/>

43. Wendie A Berg, MD, PhD, et al. *JAMA,* Vol. 397, No. 13, pp.1337-1447 LAI 4/7/12 <jama.ama-assn.org/content/307/13/1394.short>

44. Rochelle E Curtis, et al. "New Malignancies Following Breast Cancer," pp. 181-205 LAI 4/7/12 <seer.cancer.gov/publications/mpmono/Ch07_Breast.pdf>

Chapter 6

45. Department of Health and Human Services, National Institute of Allergy and Infectious Diseases, "Immune System," LAI 4/10/12 <niaid.nih.gov/topics/immunesystem/pages/default.aspx>

46. Eva Roberts, "Does Chemo Kill Yeast & Fungus?" eHow Health, LAI 4/10/12 <ehow.com/about_6686708_chemo-kill-yeast-fungus_.html>

Chapter 7

47. U.S. Food and Drug Administration, Safety, "Reclast (zoledronic acid): Drug Safety Communication – New Contradiction and Updated Warning on Kidney Impairment," LAI 4/10/12 <fda.gov/Safety/MedWatch/Safety/Information/SafetyAlertsforHumanMedicalProducts/ucm270464.htm>

48. PF Louis, "BMJ had secret financial ties to Merck during publication of articles attacking Wakefield," *Natural News,* LAI 4/10/12 <naturalnews.com/033516_BMJ_financial_ties.html>

49. Ronald Grisanti, DC, DABCO, MS, "Iatrogenic Disease: The Third Most Fatal Disease in the USA," *Your Medical Detective,* LAI 4/10/12 <yourmedicaldetective.com/public/335.cfm>

50. Maurice Hilleman, MD, "Dr. Maurice Hilleman, explains why Merck's vaccines have spread AIDS & other plagues worldwide," *YouTube,* LAI 4/10/12 <youtube.com/watch?v=4W2MJbcgn1g>

51. Miriam Rotkin-Ellman et al. "Seafood Contamination after the BP Gulf Oil Spill and Risks to Vulnerable Populations: A Critique of the FDA Risk Assessment," *Environmental Health Perspectives,* LAI 4/10/12 <ehp03.nieh.nih.gov/article/info%3Adoi%2F10.1289%2Fehp.1103695>

52. Bloomberg BusinessWeek, Archives 2006/03 Stop Soda Now, <businessweek.com/careers/workingparents/blog/archives/2006/03/stop_soda_now.html>

53. Think Before You Pink, LAI 4/10/12

Chapter 8

54. Robert Headley, "How Much Money is Spent on Cancer Research?" *Yahoo! Voices*, LAI 4/10/12 <associatedcontent.com/article/1894020/how_much_money_is_spent_on_cancer_research.html>

55. Benedict F Fitzgerald Jr, "A Report to the Senate Interstate Commerce Committee on the Need for Investigation of Cancer Research Organizations," August 3, 1953, LAI 4/10/12 <legacy.library.ucsf.edu/tid/hys5aa00/pdf>

Chapter 9

56. World Health Organization, "Ionizing Radiation," LAI 4/10/12 <who.int/ionizing_radiation/about/what_is_ir/en/index.html>

57. *The New York Times,* Health Guide, "Breast Cancer," LAI 4/10/12 <health.nytimes.com/health/guides/disease/breast-cancer/overview.html?inline=nyt-classifier>

58. National Cancer Institute, "Mammograms Key Points," LAI 4/10/12 <cancer.gov/cancertopics/factsheet/detection/mammograms>

59. Fran Lowry, "Radiation Exposure From Annual Mammography Increases Breast Cancer Risk in Young High-Risk Women," *Medscape Today News,* LAI 4/10/12 <medscape.com/viewarticle/713242>

60. Rebecca Smith-Bindman, MD, etal. "Radiation Dose Associated With Common Computed Tomography Examinations and the Associated Lifetime Attributable Risk of Cancer," *Archives of Internal Medicine,* LAI 4/10/12 <archinte.ama-assn.org/cgi/content/abstract/169/22/2078>

61. Absolute Astronomy, "Ionizing Radiation," LAI 4/10/12 <absoluteastronomy.com/topics/Ionizing_radiation>
62. YM Kirova, etal. "Radiation therapy for breast cancer increases the risk of secondary malignancy," *Nature Reviews Clinical Oncology*, August 2007, LAI 4/10/12 <nature.com/nrclinonc/journal/v4/n8/full/ncponc0872.html>
63. Jan Stejernsward, "Decreased Survival Related to Irradiation Postoperatively in Early Operable Breast Cancer," *The Lancet,* Vol. 304, Issue 7892, pp. 1285-1286, 30 November 1974, LAI 4/10/12 <thelancet.com/journals/lancet/article/PIISO140-6736(74)90142-1/abstract>
64. Chemocare.com, "Managing Chemotherapy Side Effects," LAI 4/10/12 <chemocare.com/managing/>
65. Hede, Karyn, "Chemobrain is real but may need new name," Journal of the National Cancer Institute, pp. 162-163,169, LAI 4/10/12 <jnci.oxfordjournals.org/content/early/2008/01/29/jnci.djn007.full.pdf>
66. Schilder, CM, "Cognitive functioning of postmenopausal breast cancer patients before adjuvant systemic therapy, and its association with medical and psychological factors," *Crit Rev Oncol Hematol,* 2010 Nov; 76 (2) 133-41, PubMed.gov, LAI 4/10/12 <ncbi.nlm.nih.gov/pubmed/20036141>
67. Christina M Schilder, et al. "Effects of Tamoxifen and Exemestane on Cognitive Functioning of Postmenopausal Patients With Breast Cancer: Results From the Neuropsychological Side Study of the Tamoxifen and Exemestane Adjuvant Multinational Trial," *Journal of*

Clinical Oncology, 2010, LAI 4/10/12 <jco.ascopubs.org/content/28/8/1294.full>

Chapter 10

68. Suzanne Humphries, MD, "Vaccination and Renal Patients: A Critical Examination of Assumed Safety and Effectiveness," *Vactruth.com,* October 18, 2011, LAI 4/10/12 <vactruth.com/2011/10/18/vaccination-and-renal-patients-a-critical-examination-of-assumed-safety-and-effectiveness/>

Chapter 11

69. <empr.com/increased-breast-cancer-risk-with-false-positive-test/article/235435>

70. Charles J Wright, C Barbara Mueller, "Screening mammography and public health policy: the need for perspective," *The Lancet,* July 1, 1995, Vol.346, 29-32, LAI 4/14/12 <ratical.org/radiation/Lancet7.1.95.html>

71. Pal Suhrke, PhD candidate, et al. "Effect of mammography screening on surgical treatment for breast cancer in Norway: comparative analysis of cancer registry data," *British Medical Journal,* 2011;343:d4692, LAI 4/10/12 <bmj.com/content/343/bmj.d4692.full>

72. Wikipedia, the free encyclopedia, "Mastectomy," LAI 4/10/12 <en.wikipedia.org/wiki/Mastectomy>

73. National Breast Cancer Coalition, *The Breast Cancer Deadline,* "Facts and Statistics about Breast Cancer in the United States: 2011," LAI 4/10/12 <breastcancerdeadline2020.org/know/analyses-factsheets–other/>

74. BreastCancer.org, "Genetics," LAI 4/10/12 <breastcancer.org/risk/factors/genetics.jsp>

75. Dr Frank Settle, "Nuclear Chemistry The Biological Effects of Nuclear Radiation," *Chemcases.com*, LAI 4/10/12 <chemcases.com/nuclear/nc-14.html>

76. Nora M Hansen, MD, et al. "Manipulation of the Primary Breast Tumor and the Incidence of Sentinel Node Metastases From Invasive Breast Cancer," *Archives of Surgery*, LAI 4/10/12 <archsurg.ama-assn.org/cgi/content/abstract/139/6/634>

77. Bartella, L et al. "Proton MR spectroscopy with choline peak as malignancy marker improves positive predictive value for breast cancer diagnosis: preliminary study," *Radiology*, 2006 Jun;239(3):686-92. LAI 4/10/12 <ncbi.nlm.nih.gov/sites/entrez/16603660?dopt=Abstract&holding=f1000,f1000m,isrctn>

Chapter 12

78. Pal Suhrke, PhD candidate, et al. "Effect of mammography screening on surgical treatment for breast cancer in Norway: comparative analysis of cancer registry data," *British Medical Journal*, 2011;343:d4692, LAI 4/14/12 <bmj.com/content/343/bmj.d4692.full>

79. *Wikipedia*, the free encyclopedia, "Mastectomy," LAI 4/14/12 <en.wikipedia.org/wiki/Mastectomy>

80. *National Breast Cancer Coalition*, "Facts and Statistics about Breast Cancer in the United States: 2011," LAI 4/14/12 <breastcancerdeadline2020.org/know/analyses-factsheets–other/>

81. BREASTCANCER.org, "Genetics," LAI 4/14/12 <breastcancer.org/risk/factors/genetics.jsp>

82. American Cancer Society Press Room, "New Study Says Mammography Has Little Role in Falling Breast Cancer Deaths: A Closer Look," LAI 4/14/12 <acspressroom.wordpress.com/2011/07/29/new-study-says-mammography-has-little-role-in-falling-breast-cancer-deaths-a-closer-look/>

83. Joshua A Fenton, et al. "Effectiveness of Computer-Aided Detection in Community Mammography Practice," *Journal of the National Cancer Institute,* published online July 27, 2011, LAI 4/14/12 <jnci.oxfordjournals.org/content/early/2011/07/27/jnci.djr206.abstract>

84. <assn.org/cgi/content/full/archinternmed.2011.476>

Chapter 14

85. *Prostate.Net,* "Modified Citrus Pectin – Natural Treatment for Prostate Cancer?" September 11, 2011, LAI 4/11/12 <prostate.net/2011/prevention/pectasol-c%C2%AE-modified-citrus-pectin-for-prostate-cancer/>

Chapter 15

86. Jonathan V Wright, MD, "HFCS linked to serious weight gain, liver scarring," *Dr Jonathan V Wright's Nutrition & Healing,* LAI 4/12/12 <wrightnewsletter.com/2010/04/05/hfcs-deaths/>

87. John P Pierce, PhD, et al. "Influence of a Diet Very High in Vegetables, Fruit, and Fiber and Low in Fat on Prognosis Following Treatment for Breast Cancer," *Journal of the American*

Medical Association, 2007;298(3):289-298, LAI 4/12/12 <jama. ama-assn.org/content/298/3/289.full>

88. Stephanie Meyers, MS, RD, LDN, "Does Diet Affect Cancer Recurrence?" LAI 4/12/12 <intelihealth.com/IH/ihtIH/ EMIHC268/24479/35327/593215.html?d>

Chapter 16

89a *Chemotherapyadvisor.com,* "AACR: Cruciferous Vegetable Intake Ups Breast Cancer Survival," LAI 4/9/12 <chemotherapyadvisor. com/aacr-cruciferous-vegetable-intake-ups->

89. *Quantum-Self.com,* "Protect Against Radiation Sickness," March 16, 2011, LAI 4/12/12 <quantum-self.com/quantum-library/ health-quantum-library/foods_to_protect_against_radiation_ sickness.html>

90. YouTube, "Marshall University: Walnuts and Cancer Research," LAI 4/12/12 <youtube.com/watch?v=r5dDqCS_NiA>

Chapter 17

91. *Wikipedia,* the free enclyclopedia, "Particle board," LAI 4/12/12 <en.wikipedia.org/wiki/Particle_board>

92. *Food Safety News,* "Chocolate Drink Recalled: Undeclared Wheat," LAI 4/12/12 <foodsafetynews.com/2011/08/ chocolate-drink-recalled-undeclared-wheat/>

93. *BookRags,* "Nutrition and Nutrient Transport to Cells," LAI 4/16/12 <bookrags.com/research/ nutrition-and-nutrient-transport-to-wap/>

Chapter 18

94. *cacaoweb*, "Drying and Roasting Cacao Beans," LAI 4/16/12 <cacaoweb.net/cacao-beans2.html>

95. *Grinning Planet*, "Chocolate and Pesticides / Organic Cacao," LAI 4/16/12 <grinningplanet.com/2004/02-03/pesticides-in-chocolate-organic-cocoa.htm>

96. Joy Seeman, *Digestive Health*, "Chocolate Health Benefits," LAI 4/16/12 <hemorrhoidinformationcenter.com/health-benefits-of-chololate/>

Chapter 22

97. Dr Bill Salt, "What causes free radicals in the body?" *ShareCare*, LAI 4/17/12 <sharecare.com/question/what-causes-free-radicals-body>

98. *Vaccine Excipient & Media Summary*, "Excipients Included in US Licensed Vaccines," LAI 4/17/12 <cdc.gov/vaccines/pubs/pinkbook/downloads/appendices/B/excipient-table-1.pdf>

99. Dr Packer Quotes, LAI 4/17/12 <johnpratt.com/items/docs/health/packer/quotes.html>

100. Dr Lester Packer Biography, LAI 4/17/12 <splinfo.com/lifepak_packerbio.htm>

101. Brian D Lawenda, et al. "Should Supplemental Antioxidant Administration Be Avoided During Chemotherapy and Radiation Therapy?" *Journal of the National Cancer Institute*, 2008, 100 (11):773-783, LAI 4/17/12 <jnci.oxfordjournals.org/content/100/11/773.full>

102. Kristie Leong, MD, "The Hidden Health Risks of Tea Bags," *HealthMad,* May 28, 2009, LAI 4/17/12 <healthmad.com/nutrition/the-hidden-health-risks-of-tea-bags>

103. Choice Organic Teas, "Building a Better Tea Bag," LAI 4/17/12 <choiceorganicteas.com/buildingbetterteabag.php>

Chapter 23

104. Sean Riehl, "Lymphatic Drainage Massage," *Real bodywork,* 2009, LAI 4/17/12 <deeptissue.com/articles/lymphatic_article.html>

Chapter 24

105. *University of Maryland Medical Center,* "Flaxseed oil," LAI 4/17/12 <umm.edu/altmed/articles/flaxseed-oil-000304.htm>

106. Lynn Berry, "The Health Benefits of Omega-3 in Flaxseeds," *NaturalNews,* Sept. 30, 2008, LAI 4/17/12 <naturalnews.com/024359_flax_flaxseed_omega- 3html>

107. Corsetto, PA et al. "Effects of n-3 PUFAs on breast cancer cells through their incorporation in plasma membrane," *Lipids in Health and Disease,* 2011, May 12;10:73, LAI 4/17/12 <ncbi.nlm.nih.gov/pubmed/21569413>

108. Schley, PD et al. "Mechanisms of omega-3 fatty acid-induced growth inhibition in MDA-MB-231 human breast cancer cells," LAI 4/17/12 <ncbi.nlm.nih.gov/pubmed/15986129>

Chapter 25

109. Suejung G Kim et al. "Curcumin Treatment Suppresses IKKβKinase Activity of Salivary Cells of Patients with Head and

Neck Cancer: A Pilot Study," *Clinical Cancer Research,* August 5, 2011, LAI 4/18/12 <clinicalcancers.aacrjournals.org/content/early/2011/08/05/1078-0432.CCR-11- 1272>

110. Joseph Mercola, "Cancer Cannot Thrive Without This," *LewRockwell.com,* LAI 4/18/12 <lewrockwell.com/mercola/mercola128.html>

Chapter 28

111. *Wikipedia,* the free encyclopedia, "Vitamin D," LAI 4/18/12 <en.wikipedia.org/wiki/Vitamin_D>

Chapter 29

112. *The Journal of the American Medical Association (JAMA),* "Drug Overdose Deaths—Florida, 2003-2009," 2011:306(12):1318-1320, LAI 4/18/12 <jama.ama-assn.org/content/306/12/1318.full>

113. *Alliance for Natural Health,* "Senator Durbin's Stealth Move against Supplements," October 25, 2011, LAI 4/18/12 <anh-usa.org/senator-durbin-stealth-move-against-supplements/>

Chapter 32

114. Gonzalez A, et al. "Melatonin promotes differentiation of 3T3-L1 fibroblasts," *Journal of Pineal Research,* 2012 Jan;52(1):12-20, LAI 4/18/12 <ncbi.nlm.nih.gov/pubmed/21718362>

115. Lee SE, et al. "MicroRNA and gene expression analysis of melatonin-exposed human breast cancer cell lines indicating involvement of anticancer effect," *Journal of Pineal Research,* 2011 Oct;51(3):345-52, LAI 4/18/12 <ncbi.nlm.nih.gov/pubmed/21615491>

116. Blask DE, et al. "Circadian regulation of molecular, dietary, and metabolic signaling mechanisms of human breast cancer growth by the nocturnal melatonin signal and the consequences of its disruption by light at night," *Journal of Pineal Research,* 2011 Oct;51(3):259-69, LAI 4/18/12 <ncbi.nlm.nih.gov/pubmed/21605163>

Chapter 34

117. Mike Ewall, "Bovine Growth Hormone: Milk does nobody good...," LAI 4/19/12 <ejnet.org/bgh/nogood.html>
118. *Riverside*, "Alternative cancer treatments: 11 alternative treatments to consider," MayoClinic.com Health Library, LAI 4/19/12 <riversideonline.com/health_reference/Cancer/CM00002.fm>

Chapter 37

119. Robert Preidt, "Breast Cancer Treatment Side Effects May Last for Years," *MedlinePlus,* April 11, 2012, LAI 4/21/12 <nlm.nih.gov/medlineplus/news/fullstory_123977.html>

Chapter 39

120. Ronald Grisanti, DC, DABCO, MS, "Iatrogenic Disease: The 3rd Most Fatal Disease in the USA," *Your Medical Detective,* LAI 4/21/12 <yourmedicaldetective.com/public/335.cfm>

Chapter 41

121. Kishor Gulabivala, et al. "Effects of mechanical and chemical procedures on root canal surfaces," *Endodontic Topics*

2005, 10,103-122, LAI 4/21/12 <collegeofdiplomates.
org/DrLesterQuanDVD200905/ABE%20Part%201%20
Written/Endodontic%20Topics%20%20-%20Vol%20
1%20thru%20Vol%2015Endodontic%20Topics%20
Vol%2020/,DanaInfo=www.blackwell-synergy.com+j.1601-
1546.2005.00133.pdf>

Chapter 43
122. Andrew Scholberg, "Reagan's cancer treated in Germany," LAI
4/21/12 <freegrab.net/Reagan's%20cancer%20treated%20
in%20Germany.htm>
123. American Cancer Society, Find Support & Treatment,
"Hyperbaric Oxygen Therapy," LAI 4/21/12 <cancer.org/
Treatment/TreatmentsandSideEffects/ComplementaryandAlter
nativeMedicine/HerbsVitaminsandMinerals/
hyperbaric-oxygen-therapy>

Chapter 44
124. Laura Johannes, "A Touch of Massage Therapy," *The Wall Street
Journal,* March 15, 2011, LAI 4/22/11 <online.wsj.com/article/
SB10001424052748704893604576200502111578620.html>

Chapter 45
125. Steven H Woolf, MD, MPH and Robert S Lawrence, MD,
"Preserving Scientific Debate and Scientific Choice," *Journal of
the American Medical Association (JAMA),* 1997;278(23):2105-
2108, LAI 4/22/12 <jama.ama-assn.org/content/278/23/2105.
short>

Epilogue

126. Jonathan LaPook, "Too Many Unnecessary MRIs and CT Scans?" *CBS Evening News with Scott Pelley,* September 25, 2009, LAI 4/22/12 <cbsnews.com/stories/2009/09/24/eveningnews/main5337931.shtml>

127. Sandra G. Boodman, "Concern Is Growing That The Elderly Get Too Many Medical Tests," Sep 12, 2011, *KHN/Kaiser Health News,* LAI 4/22/12 <kaiserhealthnews.org/Stories/2011/September/13/overtesting.aspx>

A Cancer Answer